Learning to care

on the
ENT WARD

Diana S Stokes
SRN, RNT

Tutor specialising
in ENT, St Bartholomew's
School of Nursing

D1744544

HODDER AND STOUGHTON
LONDON SYDNEY AUCKLAND TORONTO

LEARNING TO CARE SERIES

General Editors

JEAN HEATH, BA, SRN, SCM, CERT ED
National Health Learning Resources Unit, Sheffield
City Polytechnic

SUSAN E NORMAN, SRN, NDNCERT, RNT
Senior Tutor, The Nightingale School, West Lambeth Health Authority

Titles in this series include:

Learning to Care on the Medical Ward
A MATTHEWS
Learning to Care in the Community
P TURTON and J ORR
Learning to Care for Elderly People
L THOMAS

British Library Cataloguing in Publication Data

Stokes, D.
   Learning to care on the ENT ward. –
   (Learning to care)
   1. Otolaryngolocial nursing
   I. Title   II. Series
   617'.51'0024613   RF52.5

   ISBN 0 340 37067 X

First published 1985
Copyright © 1985 D Stokes

Typeset in 10/11 pt Trump Mediaeval
by Rowland Phototypesetting Ltd,
Bury St Edmunds, Suffolk

Printed in Great Britain for Hodder and Stoughton
Educational, a division of Hodder and Stoughton Ltd,
Mill Road, Dunton Green, Sevenoaks, Kent, by
Richard Clay (The Chaucer Press) Ltd, Bungay, Suffolk.

EDITORS' FOREWORD

In most professions there is a traditional gulf between theory and its practice, and nursing is no exception. The gulf is perpetuated when theory is taught in a theoretical setting and practice is taught by the practitioner.

This inherent gulf has to be bridged by students of nursing, and publication of this series is an attempt to aid such bridge building.

It aims to help relate theory and practice in a meaningful way whilst underlining the importance of the person being cared for.

It aims to introduce students of nursing to some of the more common problems found in each new area of experience in which they will be asked to work.

It aims to de-mystify some of the technical language they will hear, putting it in context, giving it meaning and enabling understanding.

PREFACE

Books for nurses are often written in part by doctors – this book is written by a nurse for nurses. My aims are to introduce you to the world of ear, nose and throat nursing, to interest you in the specialty, and also to try to allay some of the anxieties you may feel before entering this unfamiliar area, by discussing some of the patients you are likely to meet. Subsequently the book helps you to develop skills in problem solving, in linking theory with nursing practice and in educating for health. Today's nurses are expected to think about and critically evaluate the care they are giving, using relevant research findings; this book hopes to help you toward this challenging and new responsibility. It is intended as a reassuring introduction; a book to be used on the ward or in the department rather than selected from a library shelf.

The names used in the nursing case histories are entirely fictitious and do not refer to actual people, living or dead. The female gender is used when referring to nurses throughout, for simplicity.

I am grateful to the many medical and nursing colleagues who have given me their support so generously, to Sarah Whitfield for her thoughts, to Joan Bramley who, with endless patience, managed to decipher my notes and transform them into organised typescript and to Maggi Ansell who helped me to compile the index. I am indebted to Brian, my inspiration and mentor, to Lucy for permitting me to write and to my parents and Monica Hawkins for sharing my maternal responsibilities, which made the book become a reality.

CONTENTS

Introduction

When caring for patients with ear, nose and throat problems you will find that the general principles you have learned in other wards will apply but there are some important differences which are directly related to the nature of the specialty. Deafness, in varying degrees, is common both in children and in the elderly. When you encounter deaf people both inside the hospital and out, you need to be sensitive to the degree of sensory deprivation they are experiencing. This may be minor and the sufferer may position himself with his better hearing ear towards you, or it may lead him to feel totally isolated, as often occurs with the profoundly deaf. You will need to develop special skills in communication, and the patient will expect you to be patient, understanding and empathic.

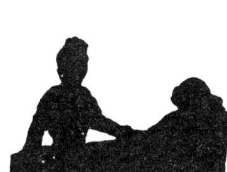

Some people you will meet may be experiencing difficulties with speech, as a result of the medical condition or the treatment being given. To help these people you will need to develop new inter-personal skills, for example you may be required to help establish an alternative method of communication.

As in the community, your patients in hospital will vary in their ethnic origin, so their language and culture will add different dimensions to your approach to their care. During your experience in this specialty you will use many of the skills you have learned in other areas but they may need some degree of adaptation to meet the needs of this different group of patients. Do remember that most patients feel anxious on visiting hospital and the way in which you approach them will be an important factor in allaying their anxiety (Franklin, 1974).

You may be apprehensive at the prospect of this new experience. When you arrive on the ward you may feel lost particularly if you do not know any of the other nurses.

You may be frightened of caring for a patient with a tracheostomy, especially if you have not seen one before. The thought of being expected to cope with a person whose tracheostomy needs suction in a hurry may worry you. This is understandable and in a caring ward environment you will be working with an experienced senior nurse who will teach you how to nurse these patients. Do use your initiative and common sense but do not be tempted to undertake, without supervision, procedures that you have not been taught. Certain procedures in ear, nose and throat nursing do carry dangers with them, for example, the tracheostomy may collapse during changing or severe bleeding may occur when nasal packing is removed, so ask to be shown how to do them safely first. When in doubt, *always ask*, but also use the care plans, the patient's notes and the procedure manuals or nursing guidelines for extra information.

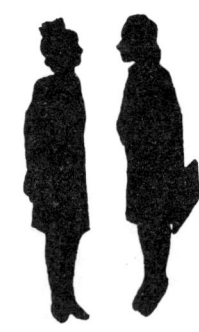

To help you become more confident, familiarise yourself early on with the emergency equipment, the suction apparatus and oxygen supply and revise the procedures for cardiac arrest and fire. Make sure you know how to operate the call system too.

Safety should always be at the back of your mind so remember to observe the procedures laid down, e.g. always use gloves when suctioning (aspirating) a tracheostomy as this protects both the patient and you against infection.

You will find great variety in ENT nursing. Your patients will range widely in age. Some may be admitted for the day only, whereas others may be with you for a long period, or need terminal care. Their problems may be minor, needing minimal care, or major, requiring skilled nursing care throughout the 24 hours. They may arrive from the Accident and Emergency Department or from the waiting list, for medical or surgical treatment. This diversity will lead you to develop differences in your approach to your patients, you will need to be sensitive to each individual situation and to react accordingly. Consequently the pace of the ward will vary from a very busy operating morning to a quiet weekend. This may feel strange to you but the quieter times do give you opportunities to get to know your patients and to learn about their care.

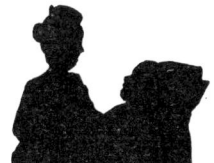

You may be doing night duty on the ward during your stay and this will require you to be especially aware of your patients and their needs during the hours of darkness. Learn to recognise the sounds of a tracheostomy requiring suction and ensure that those patients with communication difficulties have nearby a means of calling you and that they know how to use it.

This book is about *nursing*; some medical information is included but for more detail you should consult text books which are orientated towards a medical model. In the hope of catering for the wide differences in treatment and care practised across the country, some new and possibly controversial approaches have been purposely omitted. Principles of care rather than strict procedures are described so you may apply and adapt them to fit your locally agreed policies. Similarly, named drugs are not included as these will change when new ones are produced.

Each chapter contains one or more nursing histories which aim to demonstrate a holistic approach (care of the individual as a whole person. This will include not only the immediate physical or mental problem but also the concept of the person's environment, and their unique responses to their situation and state of wellness.). No one nursing model has been utilised as the choice will depend on the philosophy of your ward sister. You will see some patients appear in more than one chapter to demonstrate the continuity of care and follow their progress through various departments in the hospital. It also highlights the team approach to the care of patients as you will meet other members of the health care team who help your patient return or readjust to life outside your care.

When planning nursing care, identify the individual patient's problems from information you have gained during the assessment phase. Then with your patient you may establish the aims of that care.

'. . . a problem exists when the patient for some reason cannot meet his need' (McFarlane and Castledine, 1982). A problem may be obvious (an actual problem) or likely to occur if not prevented (a potential problem). It is important for you to realise that your personal view of your patient's needs/problems may influence your interpretation of his or her actual needs/problems. Specific nursing care (related to the particular condition) and individual care (related to the individual person) is arranged in the text using the format detailed below. General aspects of nursing care (relating to all patients) are omitted as you should be able to remember those when considering each patient. For example all patients undergoing surgery under a general anaesthetic will have the following potential problems:

CARE PLAN

Potential problem: The patient may regurgitate fluids or food during or after anaesthetic.
Nursing care and rationale: Withhold food and

fluids for four hours pre-operatively to ensure that the stomach is empty prior to the administration of the anaesthetic (Hamilton Smith, 1972).

Potential problem: Acute respiratory obstruction may occur postoperatively caused by inhalation of vomit or falling back of the tongue.
Nursing care: Nurse patient flat in a lateral position until fully awake.

At the end of each chapter there are questions which you may find useful to summarise some of the main points which have appeared in the chapter. Several ideas for further discussion with your ward sister, tutor or peers are also included and these are designed to extend your knowledge into wider issues and to introduce you to more complex nursing problems.

FURTHER READING

FRANKLIN, B. L. 1974. *Patient Anxiety on Admission to Hospital.* London: Royal College of Nursing.
HAMILTON SMITH, S. 1972. *Nil by Mouth? A Descriptive Study of Nursing Care in Relation to Pre-operative Fasting.* London: Royal College of Nursing.
MCFARLANE, J. K. & CASTLEDINE, G. 1982. *A Guide to the Practice of Nursing using the Nursing Process.* St Louis: C. V. Mosby Co.

2 Nursing in the Accident and Emergency Department

You will meet many patients who arrive in the Accident and Emergency Department with ear, nose or throat problems. Some of these problems are quickly solved in the department, whereas others necessitate admission to the ear, nose and throat ward for treatment, which may involve an operation.

The case histories of three such patients are discussed below.

HISTORY

Miss Colman has an epistaxis

Miss Colman, who is 75, arrived in the department at midday by ambulance, accompanied by her friend Mrs Lucas. She had experienced recurrent nose bleeds for 4 days but this last time the bleeding has failed to stop spontaneously. The ambulance men have unsuccessfully tried to stop the bleeding by applying digital pressure.

Miss Colman is frightened and embarrassed by the blood on her dress but the presence of her friend helps to reassure her. She is welcomed and comfortably positioned on a couch, sitting upright with her head inclined forward; a receiver and tissues are held to catch the blood. She requests that her friend remains with her and she is provided with a chair beside the couch. Miss Colman is unable to

Digital pressure

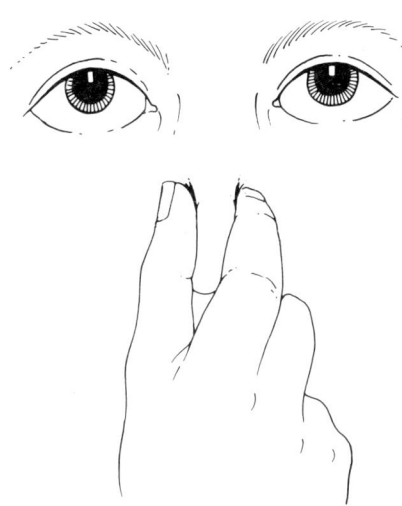

The anterior of the nose is cartilaginous and easily compressed between the thumb and first finger. Pressure is applied for 3 to 5 minutes. This may arrest the bleeding if it arises anteriorly, e.g. in Little's area, but a posterior epistaxis will not be affected by this action.

talk so with her permission Mrs Lucas answers questions and gives a brief nursing history. Miss Colman's discarded dentures are placed in a denture pot and labelled.

CARE PLAN

for Miss Colman

Actual problem: She is bleeding from her nose.
Nursing care and rationale: Nurse upright with the head inclined slightly forward to prevent backflow of blood into the pharynx, and apply digital pressure if indicated to arrest the bleeding. Record pulse, blood pressure, temperature and blood loss to assess and monitor the general condition and to detect circulatory shock. The frequency of measurements

will be determined by her condition. A receiver and tissues should be placed nearby, and soiled clothing changed to preserve her dignity.

Actual problem: She is anxious about the bleeding and treatment, admission to the department and her home situation.

Nursing care and rationale: Offer appropriate explanations for the need for the observations and treatment to lessen anxiety. Find out about any urgent home situation, deal with it and keep the patient informed of your activities and their outcome.

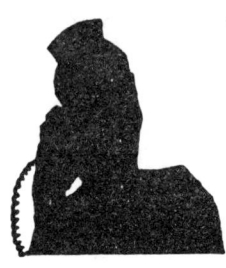

The casualty officer visits Miss Colman and having checked that she understands what is happening, he examines her nose and removes a clot from her nostril, but is unable to see the bleeding point. Following the use of a local anaesthetic spray, he inserts a nasal pack into the bleeding nostril. The nurse remains with Miss Colman and she explains the procedure, holding her hand whilst the pack is inserted.

Following this unpleasant procedure Miss Colman is comforted, offered a mouth wash and her dentures, and left to rest. She and her friend are both offered a drink. A sample of her blood is taken to measure her haemoglobin and electrolytes and for cross matching in case of further bleeding which may require a blood transfusion. In view of her age and the need to observe her carefully for further bleeding and to investigate the cause it is decided to admit her. The warden of her flat is informed by telephone. Her admission and proposed care over the next few days is discussed with them both.

In some situations patients may be sent home with nasal packing in place and return after 24 hours for its removal.

When her condition allows, she is transferred to the ward with all her belongings and medical notes, accompanied by Mrs Lucas and a nurse (see p. 23).

Nasal packing: it is usually necessary only to pack the bleeding side of the nose: bilateral bleeding is rare and blood from both sides usually means it is tracking around behind the septum. (If the bleeding vessel is identified anteriorly it may be cauterized on the spot, making packing unnecessary.) The nasal cavity is filled with 13mm ribbon gauze impregnated with an antiseptic lubricant, e.g. BIPP (bismuth, iodoform, paraffin paste). It is inserted in layers, using angled nasal forceps and Thudicum's nasal speculum, beginning on the floor of the nose and working upwards. Both ends are left visible at the external nares. An average nasal cavity will take 90–120cm of packing.

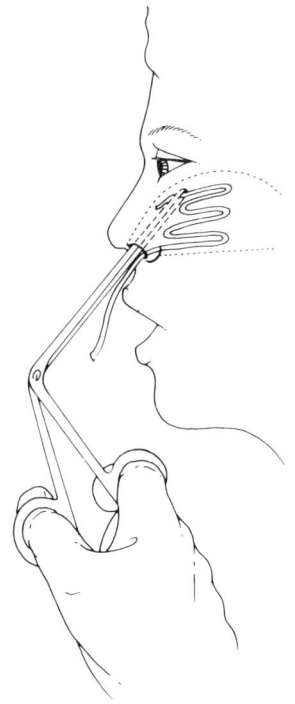

HISTORY

Steven Watts has a foreign body in his nose

Steven, aged four, arrives in the department at three in the afternoon with his mother. He has pushed a blue bead into his nose and his

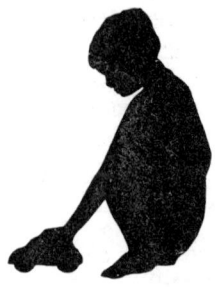

mother is worried about him; she is also concerned whether this behaviour is abnormal. They are both welcomed and Steven's toy car is admired, it runs along well on the department's floor. The nurse accompanies them to a cubicle and takes a brief nursing history. She reassures Mrs Watts that the insertion of a foreign body into the ear or nose is very common in children and is of no sinister significance. Mrs Watts appears relieved.

Foreign bodies: a wide variety of articles may be poked into ears and noses, such as beans, crayons and small pieces of toys. They may be asymptomatic until they become infected and cause discharge (otorrhoea and rhinorrhea respectively). Treatment is best left to an expert to avoid unduly distressing the child and causing further damage. Nasal foreign bodies that are lodged anteriorly may be easily removed but posterior ones may require removal under anaesthetic. Aural foreign bodies are commonly removed by syringing the ear with water, but if the ear drum is perforated, this is dangerous. Treatment should include advice against the use of cotton buds for cleaning as they may cause damage, especially if the child attempts to copy the action.

CARE PLAN

for Steven

Actual problem: He is afraid of the hospital visit.
Nursing care and rationale: Talk to and play with him to get to know him and gain his confidence; explain what is happening in terms that he can understand.

Actual problem: He has a foreign body in his nose.
Nursing care and rationale: Observe respirations for any signs of abnormality or distress, indicating that the foreign body is obstructing the airway. Help to position him on his mother's lap to facilitate examination.

The casualty officer makes friends with Steven and chats to his mother. When Steven is ready and indicates that he has understood what will happen, the doctor examines his nose with the help of a head mirror, light and Thudicum's speculum. The bead is not easily visible so Steven is referred to the ENT out-patient clinic for advice. Steven is praised for his co-operation and the plan is explained to Mrs Watts.

They are accompanied to the Outpatient Department, following a telephone call (p. 15).

Mr Harvey has swallowed a chicken bone

HISTORY

Mr Simon Harvey is 35. That day at lunch he swallowed a chicken bone which has stuck and he has been unable to swallow anything since. He is experiencing pain in his throat, but appears quite calm on admission. He is welcomed and given a comfortable seat in a cubicle, the nurse takes a brief nursing history (bearing in mind that he may have some difficulty in talking) and describes his nursing care to him. A receiver and tissues are placed beside him for his saliva. His wife is telephoned to explain what has happened and to ask her to come and give him support. They live close to the hospital.

Oesophageal obstruction by foreign body: a variety of objects may be swallowed and lodge in the pharynx or oesophagus. People wearing dentures are particularly susceptible as palatal sensation is reduced and chewing may be ineffective. Most foreign bodies lodge at the level of the crico-pharyngeus muscle and this is too low to be seen using a laryngeal mirror. Fine fish bones usually stick in the pharynx or tonsil and because of their translucency are difficult to see; they may be left to dissolve, despite the discomfort. Meat bones are dangerous because the sharp edges may perforate the oesophageal wall. Many bones are seen on lateral neck X-ray but sometimes it is necessary to perform an X-ray examination in which the patient swallows radio opaque fluid in order to identify and localise the bone. Impacted oesophageal foreign bodies usually produce acute dysphagia (difficulty in swallowing) because of the obstruction and associated muscle spasm.

for Mr Harvey

Actual problem: He is suffering acute dysphagia from the foreign body.
Nursing care and rationale: To reduce the need for swallowing and to prepare him for possible anaesthetic, offer nothing orally and place a receiver and tissues nearby.

Actual problem: He has pain in the neck at the site of the foreign body.
Nursing care and rationale: Observe the progress of the pain as analgesics may be withheld (the presence of severe pain indicates the need for urgent surgery). Record temperature, blood pressure, pulse and respirations to monitor the general condition, to detect early signs of oesophageal perforation, local surgical emphysema and mediastinitis.

Actual problem: He is anxious as a result of his admission to hospital.
Nursing care: Explain all the care and treatment to him and give appropriate reassurance.

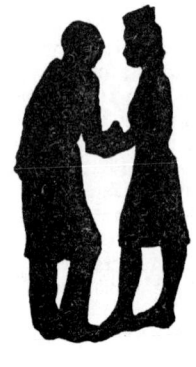

The casualty officer introduces herself to Mr Harvey and examines his mouth and larynx, using a head mirror and laryngeal mirror. The foreign body is not visible but there is pooling of saliva in the oesophagus suggesting its presence. She explains the situation to him and orders a neck X-ray (Wilson Barnett, 1978). The nurse accompanies him to the X-ray Department and takes his receiver and tissues along.

His wife arrives and is shown to a seat; her husband's care is described and her questions are answered by the doctor. Mr Harvey returns with his X-ray which shows the foreign body at the oesophageal entrance, behind the larynx. The doctor shows them the X-ray, and explains that oesophagoscopy will be necessary under general anaesthetic. She answers their questions about how long he will be in hospital. Transfer to the ward is arranged, for operation later that afternoon.

They both feel relieved that something is being done quickly and when they are ready Mr and Mrs Harvey are escorted with their belongings to the ward for his admission.

The foreign body is removed using an oesophagoscope: the complication to observe for following removal is perforation of the oesophagus leading to mediastinitis. Chest pain, rising temperature and pulse are important symptoms and should be reported early. To reduce the possibility, postoperative oral fluids are introduced gradually beginning with sterile water. If perforation has occurred, it is treated with antibiotics and diet is withheld until closure is proved.

TEST YOURSELF

1 Define epistaxis and construct a nursing care plan using the problem solving approach for a patient with an epistaxis while in the department.

2 What advice would you give to your friend whose child has put a piece of crayon into his nose/ear?

3 Where do oesophageal foreign bodies commonly lodge? What are the dangers of sharp foreign bodies in the gastro intestinal tract?

4 In what ways might you relieve the anxiety of people coming onto the Accident and Emergency Department?

5 Identify the possible problems and plan the nursing care for a patient admitted for removal of an oesophageal foreign body.

6 What additional specific nursing care would be required if the foreign body had perforated the oesophageal wall?

7 How would you recognise surgical emphysema and why does it occur?

FURTHER READING

WILSON BARNETT, J. 1978. 'Patients' emotional responses to barium X-rays.' *Journal of Advanced Nursing*, 3: 37–46.

3 Nursing in the Outpatient Department

A visit to an Outpatient Department is often the patient's first experience of hospital. As these early impressions may later affect their attitudes to care, whilst working in that department you must strive to create a non-threatening environment and one where anxieties are reduced to a minimum. You are responsible for explaining procedures and equipment in use, for ensuring the patient's comfort, reducing waiting time and facilitating communications between the doctor and patient. Three such patients visiting the department are discussed and their progress is followed.

HISTORY

Steven Watts has a foreign body in his nose

Steven, aged 4, and his mother arrive from Accident and Emergency. They are welcomed and after a short wait during which Steven plays with his toy car, they are introduced to the doctor. Steven's nursing care was outlined in Chapter 2.

The doctor makes friends slowly with Steven and tells him what he is going to do. When he is quite ready and seated on his mother's lap his nose is examined. The bead is just visible in the roof of the nose and is removed with angled forceps. Steven is praised for his co-operation and his mother is reassured. This is an ideal opportunity to talk to his mother about the general care of his nose and ears, particularly the dangers of using cotton buds. She is told that normal washing of these areas is sufficient and further interference should be avoided (the need for deeper cleaning may suggest underlying pathology which needs investigation).

Stevens does not need to come back unless Mrs Watts is worried so they leave the department and Steven waves goodbye.

HISTORY

Mrs Carter is becoming deaf

Mrs Carter is 67, with one daughter and 3 grandchildren. Her retired husband is with her and they are welcomed on arrival in the department. She was referred by her G.P. because of increasing deafness which is making her life difficult. She finds it hard to communicate with her grandchildren and is anxious not to appear 'stupid'. The nurse carefully explains what will happen to her during her visit and ensures that both she and her husband understand.

As a result of their discussion the nurse is able to identify Mrs Carter's problems and makes a plan of her care.

CARE
PLAN

for Mrs Carter

Actual problem: She has bilateral deafness; her left ear is worse than her right.
Nursing care and rationale: Spend time in communication, talking clearly and slowly and ensure that she understands. This ought to lessen the isolation she feels. Use paper and pencil if oral communication is difficult.

Actual problem: She is very anxious about the hospital visit.

Nursing care and rationale: Offer to stay with her during examinations and any planned procedures to support and give explanations.

Mr and Mrs Carter are shown into the doctor's room and made comfortable. A full medical history is taken which includes details of the degree of disability Mrs Carter is experiencing and how it has changed her life. On examination of her ears they are found to contain impacted wax so the nurse is requested to syringe them before hearing testing may proceed.

Mrs Carter is taken to another room and comfortably positioned in an upright chair. The nurse carefully explains the procedure and answers Mrs Carter's questions. Her husband is invited to stay with her to support her.

Ear Syringing

Protect clothing
Inspect ear with otoscope
Hold pinna upwards to straighten canal and *support* syringe
Exclude air from syringe and direct water onto posterior/superior canal wall, the patient holds receiver under ear
Inspect again
Dry mop canal

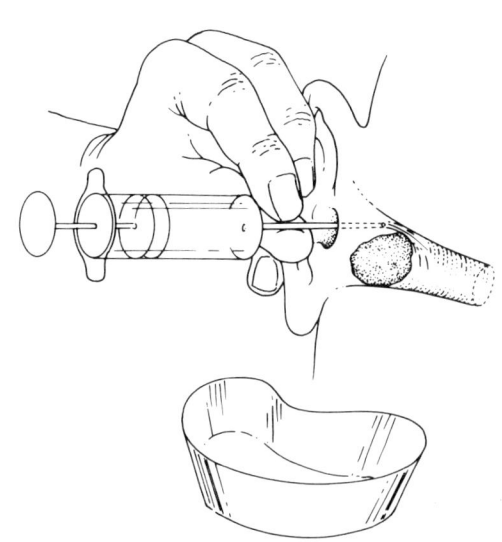

Syringing may also be used to remove debris in otitis externa. It carries with it the dangers of perforation of the tympanic membrane and so should only be performed by an experienced practitioner. Care should be taken to ensure that there is no existing perforation as the patient may feel dizzy and infection may be introduced into the middle ear.

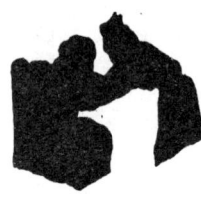

Mrs Carter is encouraged to rest for a short while and have a cup of tea prior to returning to the doctor (sometimes it is better for the patient to go home and return the next week for the rest of the investigations, particularly if she has been distressed by this procedure).

The doctor continues to examine Mrs Carter's ears, nose and throat using illumination and tests her hearing with a tuning fork.

She then has an audiogram performed to further assess her hearing loss, and this procedure is carefully explained. She is taken into the sound proof room.

Pure tone audiometry: sounds at varying frequencies (measured in Hertz, Hz) and of differing intensities are delivered to each ear independently and the threshold (the lowest intensity of sound which can be heard) is recorded in decibels (dB). Both air conduction and bone conduction are measured and plotted on a chart.

When Mrs Carter returns to the doctor with her results accompanied by her husband, the complete situation is explained to her. She has a bilateral sensori-neural loss which is worse in her left ear. The cause of this is presbycusis (degenerative changes associated with ageing) and will be best helped by using a hearing aid. Her subsequent management is described; she will have a hearing aid fitted by the audiometrician and a programme of instruction planned by the hearing therapist.

They are both relieved that the cause of deafness has been found and that no operation is necessary. Mrs Carter is keen to try a hearing aid so she can hear her grandchildren talking again. She is given an appointment for the fitting and leaves the department happily.

Normal audiogram

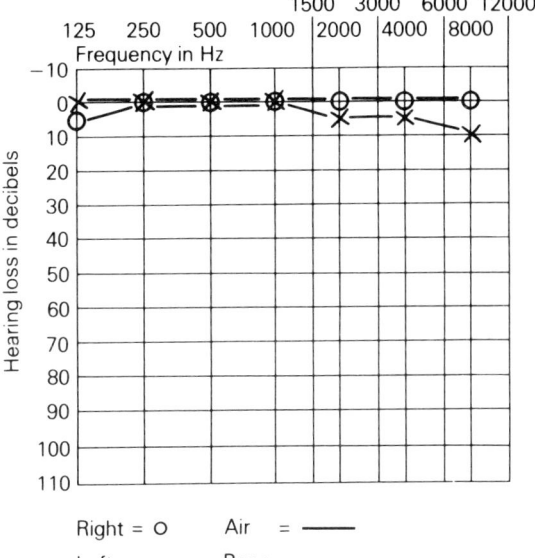

Sensori-neural deafness in presbycusis

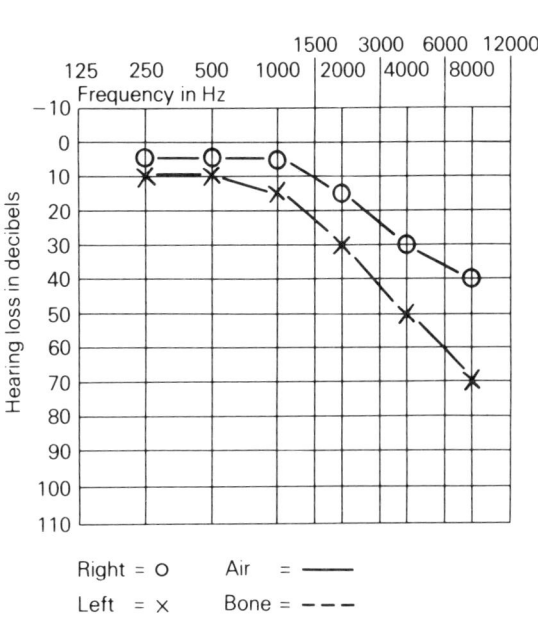

Mr Andrews has otitis externa

Mr Andrews, a 50 year old insurance agent, arrives in the department for his ear dressing. He has chronic otitis externa and is being treated with daily dressings to the auditory canal. He tells the nurse that he cannot hear very well and is worried about this.

Otitis externa: infections of the external ear may be caused by bacterial or fungal invasion of the epithelium. This causes pain, swelling and aural discharge accompanied sometimes by some loss of hearing and lymphadenopathy (enlargement of the lymph nodes). Treatment of the acute form includes analgesics, local heat application, gentle cleansing of the canal and instillation of antibiotic drops or an impregnated gauze wick. Ear drops (at room temperature) are instilled by pulling the pinna upward and backward, with the head tilted towards the unaffected side. In chronic otitis externa pain is uncommon but itching is frequently experienced. The canal may be dry and scaly. Here the canal is cleansed and a wick impregnated with antibiotic (often accompanied by a steroid) ointment inserted daily until the condition improves. Skin disorders such as psoriasis and seborrhoeic dermatitis may also be associated with otitis externa.

He is welcomed, shown in to the treatment room and comfortably positioned on a chair. His problem is identified and care planned. As this is the second day of his treatment he is no longer anxious about the procedure and the care plan remains the same. He says the discomfort is less.

CARE PLAN

for Mr Andrews

Actual problem: He is suffering from itching in his external auditory canal due to the chronic otitis externa.

Nursing care and rationale: Inspect the canal using an otoscope after removing the old gauze wick. Gently cleanse the canal using 'fluffed' cotton wool loaded on an applicator or Jobson

Horne probe to remove discharge. (Commercially prepared ones are too large and too firm to absorb discharge.) Inspect again and carefully insert 1cm wide impregnated gauze dressing using angled forceps, feeding it in little by little to ensure the whole canal is filled. This should lessen the itching. Protect his clothing during this procedure to prevent soiling from the discharge and thus preserving his dignity.

The procedure should be carried out by an experienced practitioner to avoid damage to the canal or tympanic membrane.

Mr Andrews is reassured that the deafness caused by the dressing is only temporary and he is advised to refrain from touching his ears, allowing water in or poking articles inside as these may re-infect the canal. He is told that when the condition is cured, simple washing of the outer ear with soap and water and thorough drying is all it requires.

He leaves the department more comfortable and is requested to return the following day to repeat the procedure.

TEST
YOURSELF

1 How would you ensure that a patient's first visit to this hospital department was a happy one?

2 What information would you give to:
The mother of a child with a foreign body in his nose.
A teenager about the cleaning of her ears.
A junior nurse watching you syringe a patient's ears.

3 Many nasal conditions are associated with allergy and part of the care involves investigating the cause of the allergy. Try to visit the clinic and find out how these tests are performed and what advice the patient is subsequently given.

4 Patients who complain of vertigo are investigated using the Caloric test. How is the test performed and the results interpreted? What effect does the test have on the patient and what nursing care will be required?

5 Discuss electronystagmography with the outpatient sister in relation to the preparation, support and explanation the patient will need.

6 What other tests (including tuning fork tests) are regularly performed in the department? How do they affect the patient?

4 Nursing Miss Colman with an epistaxis

HISTORY

Miss Colman is a 75 year old lady who lives on her own on the ground floor of a small block of flats supervised by a warden. She has no family but her devoted friend Mrs Lucas, a widow, lives next door to her. She has an elderly cat called Ginger, she listens to the radio with interest and when collected attends her local church on Sunday mornings.

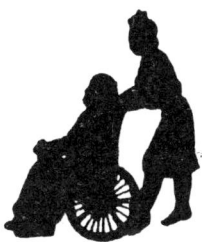

A thin frail lady, she has had recurrent nose bleeds for four days and her neighbour called an ambulance to take her to the Accident and Emergency Department for investigation. After her nose is packed and blood is taken for haemoglobin, electrolytes and cross matching, she is transferred to the ward in a wheelchair, accompanied by her friend.

Epistaxis: epistaxis or nose bleeding is a common condition mostly arising from the anterior part of the nasal septum where there is a plexus of tiny arteries and veins. Less frequently, bleeding comes from the posterior of the nose (anterior ethmoidal and maxillary arteries). This is more common in the elderly and may be severe, even life-threatening.

Causes

Local	*General*
'Spontaneous'	Cardiovascular
Trauma	(e.g. hypertension)
Atrophic rhinitis	Blood vessel
Tumours of nose	abnormality
or sinuses	Blood disorders
Hereditary telangiectasia	(e.g. leukaemia)
	Vitamin K deficiency

An anterior epistaxis is usually easily controlled by local pressure whereas a posterior one is more difficult to stop as the offending vessel is out of sight and bleeding is often more profuse.

Initial stages

Miss Colman and Mrs Lucas are welcomed and after Miss Colman has been settled comfortably sitting up in bed on a sheepskin where she may be easily observed, her problems are identified.

Using the information from her nursing assessment they plan her care together, and the nurse gives a full explanation of the situation. Miss Colman shows immediate concern for Ginger and Mrs Lucas offers to look after him and to inform the warden of the current situation. The nurse checks the bedside radio, light and communication buzzer to ensure they are working correctly.

for Miss Colman

Actual problem: She is still bleeding from her nose.

Nursing care and rationale: Record pulse, blood pressure and fluid balance to detect circulatory shock from loss of blood. Observe for nasal bleeding through nasal pack and apply a nasal bolster to catch any oozing, changing it as necessary. Administer a mild sedative as prescribed if she is overactive and analgesics for relief of nasal discomfort. Leave a receiver and tissues nearby.

Actual problem: She is confined to bed to help prevent further bleeding and may suffer pressure sores, deep vein thrombosis, chest infection and constipation (complications of immobilisation) if these are not prevented by appropriate nursing intervention.

Nursing care and rationale: Nurse sitting upright until the nasal pack is removed and bleeding has ceased to prevent backflow of blood into the pharynx. Offer the commode

Occasionally a severe epistaxis will lead to circulatory shock and the patient's care will be planned accordingly. Intravenous fluids would be indicated and if the haemoglobin is below 10g/dl blood transfusion is likely to be necessary. The nursing observations are carried out according to local practice.

regularly to encourage elimination. Give assistance with washing to meet personal hygiene needs. Offer frequent mouth washes to prevent drying because of mouth breathing.

Nasal bolster in place

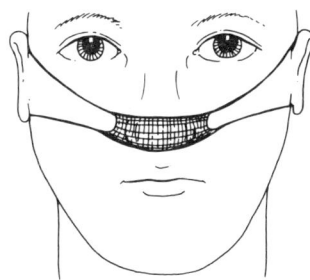

During her two days in bed Miss Colman receives a visit from her local vicar and Mrs Lucas comes in regularly with clean night clothes and news of Ginger.

After 48 hours her nasal packing is removed by a senior nurse. Miss Colman sits up in bed with her clothes protected and holds a receiver under her chin. The nurse explains the procedure as she is working and although it feels unpleasant, Miss Colman says the relief afterwards is worth it. She rests in bed for a while and a new nasal bolster is applied.

If bleeding continues despite anterior nasal packing a posterior nasal pack may be used as well. This will be of the gauze type or inflatable e.g. Brighton balloon, which exerts pressure in the nose both anteriorly and posteriorly.

In the unlikely event that these do not stop the bleeding surgical intervention may be indicated in the form of ligation of the offending artery.

Brighton balloon

As no fresh bleeding is seen Miss Colman is encouraged to get up and gradually resume normal activities until she feels strong enough to go home.

Evaluation

Regular reassessment of her care reveals no complications and discharge home is planned. Meanwhile the cause of her nosebleed is investigated; as she is not found to be hypertensive and no local pathology is found on her sinus X-rays, the cause is probably due to friable blood vessels and therefore may recur. This is all explained to Miss Colman, and both she and her neighbour are instructed in her care should it happen again.

The haemoglobin level is again estimated and, as it is low, oral iron is prescribed. This is also explained to them both and the importance of continuing the tablets is stressed. Miss Colman is tactfully told of its side effects (constipation and blackening of the stools) and she is advised to include more roughage in her diet to help prevent constipation.

Planning discharge

Although tired Miss Colman feels well and is anxious to get back to Ginger, so transport home is arranged and the warden informed. Mrs Lucas has prepared the flat and bought some groceries for her and Ginger. Miss Colman is advised to take life easily for a while, avoiding lifting and nose blowing as this increases venous pressure. A follow up outpatient appointment and transport are arranged for one month later and her G.P. is informed of her stay in hospital.

1 What are the causes of epistaxis?

2 What problems does a patient with an epistaxis experience?

3 Construct a nursing care plan for the first 48 hours in the ward.

4 How would you prepare the patient for discharge and what advice would you give?

5 Consider the additional problems to be faced by a patient who was admitted in a shocked condition following severe epistaxis.

6 Occasionally the bleeding is relentless and surgery is indicated to save life; how will this affect your care?

5 Nursing patients with infections

Upper respiratory tract infections are common in both adults and children. The mucous membrane forms a continuous lining throughout the tract and into the middle ear so that spread of infection into other areas is common. Most of these patients are cared for by the G.P. at home. The following case histories are of patients with conditions, although not common, that warrant hospital admission.

Terry Wild has a quinsy

Terry Wild is a 23 year old unemployed building labourer who lives with his mother in a council flat. He is tall, plump and on arrival from the Accident and Emergency Department appears unshaven and ill. He has suffered from recurrent attacks of tonsillitis in the past; the present attack began one week ago. He now has severe pain in his throat, is unable to swallow even his saliva or to open his mouth very widely, his voice is muffled and he feels feverish. He has no G.P. so he came to the Accident and Emergency Department where the diagnosis of quinsy was made.

Quinsy (peritonsillar abscess): peritonsillar abscess usually follows acute tonsillitis. An abscess develops between the tonsil capsule and the lateral pharyngeal wall causing a unilateral swelling which may obscure the tonsil and displacing the uvula across the midline.

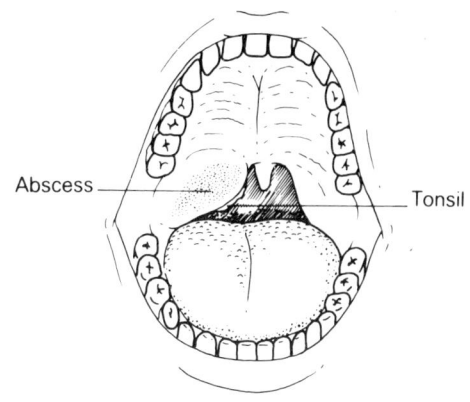

Abscess — Tonsil

The presenting signs and symptoms include pyrexia, pain, difficulty with swallowing, intense salivation, trismus (reflex masseteric muscle spasm), halitosis, thickened speech and cervical lymphadenopathy. Conservative treatment involves giving large doses of antibiotics intravenously. Non-resolution or respiratory distress from the swelling necessitates incision of the abscess. Great care is necessary to protect the airway during this procedure. Tonsillectomy may be indicated at a later date to prevent recurrence.

NURSING CARE

Initial stages

Terry (he prefers to be addressed by his first name) is welcomed and accompanied to his bed. He is given light cotton pyjamas, a dressing gown and toilet articles as he arrived unprepared for admission. A nurse helps him into bed and makes him comfortable, placing a receiver and tissues nearby. She takes a brief nursing history although as he is finding speech painful only essential questions are asked. A message is sent to his mother via a neighbour's telephone to request her to bring him any belongings he may need. The doctor examines him, takes a specimen of blood and a throat swab. An intravenous infusion is sited and fluids are commenced to prevent de-hydration.

A nurse explains each step to him but he feels too unwell to ask questions. Having ascertained that he has no antibiotic allergies, intravenous antibiotic therapy is commenced. His nursing problems are identified and his care planned.

CARE PLAN

for Terry

Actual problem: He is suffering severe pain in the throat.
Nursing care and rationale: Observe for pain and control it by administering analgesics as prescribed. Monitor their effectiveness.

Actual problem: He has pyrexia as a result of the abscess.
Nursing care and rationale: Record observations of pulse, temperature and respirations to monitor his general condition and report any changes that could indicate complications, such as a rigor or septicaemia. Nurse him in light cotton clothing and tepid sponge or fan him if indicated to reduce his temperature. Change the damp clothing frequently to maintain comfort.

Actual problem: He has difficulty in swallowing and therefore is not able to drink adequately while losing considerable fluids from sweating.
Nursing care and rationale: Place receiver and tissues nearby to spit unswallowed saliva into and offer frequent oral hygiene to prevent mouth infection. Ensure that the intravenous line is patent so that fluids can be administered as prescribed to maintain hydration. Observe the infusion site frequently to detect local inflammation and infection. Offer oral fluids when he can swallow and encourage a progression to a normal diet.

Actual problem: He is anxious about his condition and hospital admission.

Nursing care and rationale: Offer brief explanations (as he feels unwell) of all his treatment and nursing care. Discuss and deal with any social problems he might have.

Terry's mother comes to visit him and his condition and care are discussed with them both. She is reassured that he is improving and will soon be discharged. His temperature returns to normal and his pain lessens after two days and he begins to swallow. When he is taking adequate amounts of fluids orally his intravenous infusion is discontinued and antibiotics are given orally in suspension form. He increases his activities and looks after himself. He is getting bored so he is introduced to the hospital library and television room. His bedside radio is checked, and he is shown how to use it.

NURSING CARE

Evaluation

Regular reassessments of the nursing aims and Terry's progress reveal that he has developed no further complications, and plans for his discharge are made.

NURSING CARE

Planning discharge

He is advised to register with a G.P. on discharge and visit his dentist for a check-up. (Quinsy may be associated with poor dental hygiene.) A nurse tactfully teaches him measures to prevent dental decay and gives him information regarding his diet in the hope that he will be encouraged to reduce his weight. He is given the remainder of his antibiotics to take home and the importance of completing the course is heavily stressed. Although unemployed now, he is searching for work and is told he will need to take two weeks' convalescence before he commences. In view of the plan to proceed to tonsillectomy in six weeks' time he decides to postpone working until after the operation, so he does not need to take sick leave immediately after beginning a new job. The details of the proposed operation are discussed and he is asked to return in one month for a check-up in outpatients.

HISTORY

Miss Pearl Hunt has frontal sinusitis

Pearl is a 19 year old student nurse from Jamaica. Her parents are still in the West Indies but she has an older brother who lives with his family near her training school. Her main interests are reading and popular music.

Pearl is admitted at her G.P.'s request with an acute frontal sinusitis. She had a cold a week ago and is now complaining of severe frontal headache, swelling of her right eyelid (orbital cellulitis), which has closed her eye, and malaise. Normally tall, slim and healthy, she now looks ill with a temperature of 40°C.

Sinusitis: sinusitis is a suppurative infection in one or more of the paranasal sinuses.

It may be acute or chronic and often follows infective rhinitis or is associated with an allergic reaction. The signs and symptoms are pain and tenderness over the affected sinus, nasal obstruction, loss of smell, malaise and pyrexia. The condition is diagnosed by X-ray which shows the sinus to be opaque, containing purulent fluid rather than air.

Untreated sinusitis can lead to serious complications as a result of the proximity of the sinuses to the brain. Amongst these are: frontal lobe abscess, meningitis, cavernous sinus thrombosis, septicaemia and osteomyelitis. Initial treatment is usually conservative with antibiotics and sometimes the use of a decongestant nasal spray to aid drainage. If this fails and acute symptoms persist the sinus is drained surgically. Chronic sinusitis produces less severe symptoms but on X-ray, fluid may be seen and the mucous membrane lining is thickened. Treatment is by antrum puncture and wash-out of the sinus, or by intranasal antrostomy and making a permanent opening into the nose below the inferior turbinate bone.

NURSING CARE

Initial stages

Pearl arrives on the ward accompanied by her boy friend Colin, they are welcomed and shown to her bed. When she is comfortably scttled in bed, the bathrooms and toilets are pointed out for her use whenever she feels able to get up. A nursing history is taken by the nurse and her boy friend helps to clarify some of the answers for her. Colin suggests that he should contact Pearl's brother who could telephone their parents, calmly explaining the situation. After the doctor's examination in the presence of the nurse, her condition and treatment are fully discussed with Pearl and Colin. She has worked on an ear, nose and throat ward so she understands what is involved, but she does not feel well enough to help plan her own care. The doctor explains that he will examine the affected eye frequently and should her vision be threatened, an operation to drain the abscess will be necessary. She has no antibiotic allergies so an intravenous cannula is inserted into the back of her left hand (she is right-handed) and antibiotics are commenced. The antibiotics are administered intravenously to introduce a high level quickly in the body as the abscess is close to the brain and may spread. A specimen of blood is taken for examination including that for sickle cell disease. Pearl's problems are identified and her care is planned.

for Pearl

Actual problem: She has a severe frontal headache from the sinusitis.
Nursing care and rationale: Administer prescribed analgesics to help control the pain. Monitor their effectiveness.

Actual problem: She has a high temperature as a result of the infection.
Nursing care and rationale: Record observations of temperature and pulse to monitor condition and detect complications. Nurse her with frequent changes of cool clothing. To prevent dehydration offer her at least three litres of her choice of fluids per day.

Actual problem: Her right eye is closed due to orbital cellulitis.
Nursing care and rationale: Observe the affected eye and monitor the swelling for any changes. Bathe it as necessary using sterile 0.9% saline and an aseptic technique to keep the area clean and increase comfort. The abscess may damage the optic nerve, reducing vision.

Actual problem: She is very anxious about her condition and whether it will affect her training.
Nursing care and rationale: Offer her detailed explanations of her care and treatment. Communicate with the school of nursing to reassure her about her future.

Actual problem: She has an intravenous cannula in her hand which may become blocked or displaced or the site of insertion may become infected.
Nursing care and rationale: Observe the cannula and the site regularly.

The next morning when Pearl's vision is assessed by the doctor, she reports some deterioration so an urgent operation is planned. The nature of this is discussed with her, and her brother is informed. She is quickly prepared and accompanied to the operating theatre.

When her condition is satisfactory after the operation she returns to the ward. She has a small incision beside the inner canthus of the eye and a silastic drainage tube has been inserted to drain pus from her frontal sinus into her nose.

The facial wound

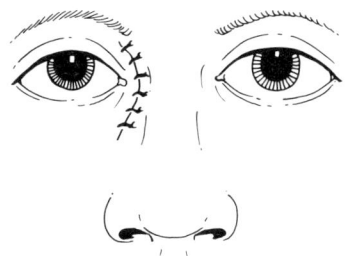

<table>
<tr><td>CARE PLAN</td></tr>
</table>

for Pearl postoperatively

Actual problem: She has a facial wound.
Nursing care and rationale: Observe the wound for bleeding and infection. Give her frequent clean nasal bolsters for the oozing. Remove sutures aseptically when the wound has healed.

Pearl's general condition and eyelid swelling improve dramatically and she is out of bed and beginning to listen to her favourite music on her radio headphones. She is advised not to blow her nose as this may reinfect the sinus or infect the orbit. Her antibiotics are continued orally and the intravenous cannula is removed from her hand.

Evaluation

Regular evaluation of her care confirms her improvement. Colin and her brother visit regularly and are very pleased to see this.

Planning discharge

Arrangements are made for her discharge; she will go and convalesce at her brother's as his wife can look after Pearl for a fortnight until she is able to return to work.

The doctor explains that the drainage tube should remain inside her nose for 4 to 6 weeks and she is given an outpatient appointment. She readily accepts this as she can neither see nor feel the tube in her nose. She has completed the course of antibiotics and thus does not need to take any home.

On leaving the ward Pearl says she feels better equipped now to nurse her own patients, having experienced a spell in hospital herself.

1 What is a peritonsillar abscess and what are the predisposing features?

2 What are the complications of the condition and how would you recognise them?

3 Describe sinusitis, how it affects a person and the possible complications.

4 What safety precautions would you take if a patient's peritonsillar abscess was to be incised on the ward under local anaesthetic?

5 What nursing problems does the operation, antral washout and antrostomy pose, and what might your nursing aims be?

6 Consider the additional nursing care required if the sinus infection leads to meningitis.

6 Nursing Mr Mitchell who is undergoing nasal surgery

Nasal obstruction is a common complaint caused by mechanical displacement (as by fracture) of the nasal bones or as a result of disorders which cause swelling of the nasal mucous membranes (e.g. allergic rhinitis). One such condition and its care will be discussed and any significant differences relating to the other common operations will be highlighted at the end of the chapter.

HISTORY

Mr Mitchell is a 40 year old accountant, married with twin boys aged 10. He lives in a large house in the country and commutes daily to work. His main interest is sport; he played rugby for his county until 10 years ago when he took up squash. He plays three times a week at his local club. He does not smoke and only drinks socially. His G.P. referred him to the outpatients for investigation of a unilateral nasal obstruction. On examination, he was found to have a deflected nasal septum, as a result of an old nasal injury.

Admission was advised for *submucous resection* of the septum to restore his airway.

Submucous resection: deformity of the nasal septum is common, indeed it is rarely straight, but if it is very deflected as a result of injury, it causes nasal obstruction.

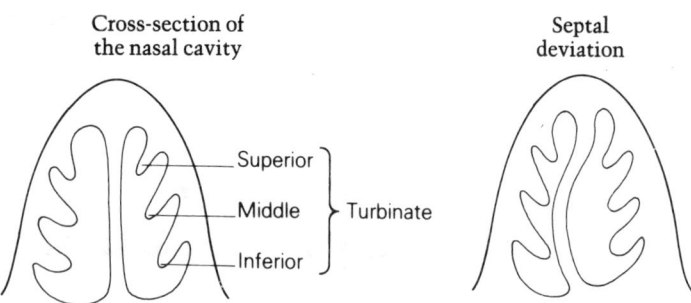

Cross-section of
the nasal cavity

Septal
deviation

Superior ⎤
Middle ⎬ Turbinate
Inferior ⎦

Treatment is by removing the obstructing cartilage and
with the aid of bilateral nasal packing, the
mucoperichondrial flaps are held straight in the midline.
The operation may be done under general or local
anaesthesia. In order to reduce mucosal oedema and
bleeding, the nose is packed with 13mm ribbon gauze
soaked (not dripping) in equal quantities of Cocaine 10%
and Adrenaline 1 in 1000 pre-operatively.

NURSING CARE

Initial stages

Mr Mitchell, a tall, fit-looking man, arrives on
the ward with his wife. They are both welcomed by a nurse and shown around the ward.
When they are settled and his belongings are
unpacked, a nursing history is taken prior to
the doctor's examination. The operation and
length of stay are discussed with them both
and visiting times are planned, so that the
twins may be able to come too. Mr Mitchell
appears relaxed and confident and says he is
looking forward to the rest. He helps the nurse
to identify his pre-operative problems and plan
his care.

CARE PLAN

for Mr Mitchell pre-operatively

Actual problem: He has a blocked right nostril
and this discomfort may prevent him sleeping
well.

Nursing care and rationale: Allocate him a bed

in a well-ventilated part of the ward and offer prescribed sedation if necessary.

After Mr Mitchell is given his pre-medication his nose is packed by an experienced nurse with cocaine and adrenaline soaked ribbon gauze. (Occasionally a patient may become pale and sweaty with low blood pressure as a result of cocaine absorption.) The procedure is carefully explained to him and he co-operates well. A nurse accompanies him to the operating theatre, talking to him during the journey. Following the operation, when his condition is stable, he is transferred to the ward and his postoperative care is planned.

| CARE PLAN | for Mr Mitchell postoperatively |

Actual problem: His nose is packed with BIPP impregnated ribbon gauze, which may cause pain and insomnia and lead to anorexia and a dry mouth due to the necessity to mouth breathe.
Nursing care and rationale: Observe for any bleeding through the packing and apply a nasal bolster as necessary, changing it when required to preserve his dignity. Offer oral fluids frequently and administer prescribed sedatives and analgesics as necessary.

Mr Mitchell is soon out of bed and looking after himself. He complains of a sucking action in his throat as he swallows, he is told that this is quite normal and is a result of the packing in the nose causing a partial vacuum in the throat on swallowing. His family visits him regularly. He is experiencing a small amount of serous discharge from his nose but otherwise feels well.

After 24 hours his packing is removed. The procedure is explained to him and he sits up-

Occasionally there may be prolonged brisk bleeding which necessitates repacking by the surgeon.

right in bed with his clothing protected, holding a receiver under his chin. The gauze is removed slowly and he has a small amount of bleeding which quickly stops spontaneously. A fresh nasal bolster is applied.

He is asked to rest in bed for a short while, to avoid bending his head forward or blowing his nose (the latter for 2 weeks).

NURSING CARE

Evaluation

Reassessment of his nursing care reveals no complications. He has no signs of septal haematoma or infection.

When his family visits, his progress is obvious and they are pleased to hear that they may take him home the following day.

NURSING CARE

Planning discharge

As Mr Mitchell prepares to go home he is again advised not to blow his nose and to wait 3 weeks before recommencing squash. These precautions are to ensure that the muco-perichondrial flaps do not separate leading to the development of a septal haematoma. He has planned to take a fortnight's leave to recuperate and is given an outpatient appointment on leaving.

Other conditions commonly found

Nasal polypectomy. People with allergic rhinitis (nasal allergy) frequently have nasal polyps. They are pale, soft translucent masses of oedematous stroma covered by mucous membrane. They are usually multiple and bilateral and originate from the ostia or from within the sinus itself. The allergy is investigated and then treatment is by removal under local or general anaesthesia, but they frequently recur. The nursing problems and nursing care are similar to those mentioned above.

Fractured nasal bones. Fracture of the nasal bones may result from a wide variety of injuries. If no external displacement or airway obstruction is apparent, no treatment is necessary. If external or internal deformity results, surgical reduction of the fracture is indicated. This is ideally undertaken before 10 days have passed or poor union will have started. The fracture is reduced under local or general anaesthesia and the unstable bones are supported in their correct position by an external plaster of Paris splint and internal nasal packing. The packing is removed after 24 hours but the splint remains for 10 days, care being taken that pressure sores are not developing underneath. The nursing care is again similar to that discussed above. Bear in mind that the patient may be very worried about permanent disfigurement. The patient is advised to prevent any repeated injury until the fracture has united.

| TEST YOURSELF |

1 What are the common causes of nasal obstruction?

2 What are the specific problems facing a patient who has undergone nasal surgery to improve the airway?

3 Discuss the complications and the means by which you would recognise them.

4 Consider the additional problems and the nursing care required by a patient having his operation performed under local anaesthesia.

7 Nursing children

Children in Hospital

Children, as do most adults, prefer to be nursed at home when they are ill. Thus if a child needs to be admitted to hospital, care should be taken to provide as homely an environment for the whole family as possible. Wherever possible the parent should be encouraged to be resident with the child, and unrestricted visiting should be the ward policy (Ministry of Health, 1959). If parents are not able to visit, you must then realise your role as a parent substitute (Hawthorn, 1974).

In order to look after a child you should try to understand how he or she feels. He may have some ideas about hospitals from the television but in reality, uniforms and equipment may be frightening. Indeed hospitalisation may have been used as a threat to the child, so he may view the experience as punishment and some treatments administered in hospital could easily reinforce that view. It is important for you to be aware that children are admitted at different stages of development and independence and of varying cultural and social backgrounds. All these aspects must be considered when you are assessing the child's needs and planning individual care.

If a child has been emotionally prepared before entering hospital, he settles more readily and is more co-operative in his care and treatment (Which? 1980). This is not always possible with an emergency admission but for planned spells in hospital a variety of ideas may be used including role play, stories and ward visits. The family's Health Visitor will help in this preparation, providing a useful link between hospital and home. Another very important point is to provide both parent and child with honest information, compatible with his or her individual level of understanding.

You need to be aware of the parents' anxiety and try to involve them in the child's care, taking note of their judgement of the child's condition where offered. Involvement may also be extended to other siblings and this may avoid jealousy over the increased attention being received by the ill member of the family.

A large proportion of the treatments for ear, nose and throat conditions in children involve surgery. Although stay is usually short, an anaesthetic and an operation increases the anxiety felt by both the parent and the child.

When working on the children's ward the following children are likely to be encountered. One child's care is discussed in detail followed by brief information on others, highlighting important differences.

HISTORY

Charlotte is the seven year old only child of professional parents. She has been absent from school frequently during the past year with attacks of acute tonsillitis, one of which was complicated by otitis media. Her G.P. referred her to the ear, nose and throat outpatients where it was decided to remove her tonsils and adenoids. Charlotte's last attack of tonsillitis occurred 4 weeks before admission.

Tonsils and Adenoids: the tonsils and adenoids form part of a circular band of lymphoid tissue surrounding the entrance to the respiratory tract. The adenoids (nasal pharyngeal tonsils) lie in the roof and wall of the nasopharynx and are best developed in childhood. They are closely applied to the opening of the pharyngo-tympanic (Eustachian) tube which accounts for the spread of infection to the middle ear. The tonsils have crypts (deep recesses) over their surfaces and are situated in the lateral walls of the oropharynx.

Tonsillitis: tonsillitis is caused by various microorganisms (e.g. haemolytic streptococcus) and is characterised by fever, pain in the throat, reluctance to swallow, swollen, inflamed tonsils with yellow exudate arising from the crypts and enlarged, tender cervical lymph glands. Complications include otitis media, quinsy, acute glomerular nephritis and rheumatic fever. Treatment is initially conservative with antibiotics and analgesics. Operative treatment is no longer fashionable but frequent absence from school is one criterion which might justify removal of the child's tonsils. Surgery carries a very small mortality rate but should not be embarked upon without justification.

Charlotte's parents have carefully prepared her for admission; they have explained what will happen with the use of the hospital booklet, a story book and playing 'hospitals'. Charlotte and her mother visit the ward before admission to help allay their anxieties and familiarise Charlotte with the ward and its occupants.

<table>
<tr><td>NURSING
CARE</td></tr>
</table>

Initial stages

Charlotte and her mother are welcomed by a nurse and are shown to her bed. Her mother has arranged to remain with her daughter and is given a bed next to her (this is not always possible). After they have unpacked they are again given a tour of the ward which includes the facilities for resident parents. Charlotte has brought in her teddy bear called Ben and a picture of the ward she painted at home and this is put on the wall by her bed. They are told who the nurses, doctors and domestic staff are and Charlotte writes their names on her picture. When both appear settled, the nurse takes a nursing history and gives both Charlotte and Ben identity bands to wear. The doctor makes friends with Charlotte and examines her. He explains why he needs to take a blood sample and after Ben has had his 'prick', Charlotte agrees to have hers. They talk about the operation and Charlotte asks what she will be able to eat afterwards. Mrs Evans signs the consent form when she is sure she understands all that is involved. Using the information gathered, the nurse plans Charlotte's care together with her mother.

CARE PLAN

for Charlotte pre-operatively

Actual problem: She is anxious after coming into hospital.

Nursing care and rationale: Gain her confidence by playing with her. Offer her and her mother honest appropriate explanations of all treatments and nursing care and relate it to the books she has read. Ensure that her mother is familiar with the facilities provided for resident parents which are aimed at producing a homely environment.

Charlotte is carefully prepared for operation with her mother's help. She is given a drink 6 hours before the operation (Hamilton Smith, 1972) and all her sweets and drinks are removed from the locker. Her mother offers to ensure nothing is taken orally. Charlotte's teeth are checked to ensure none are loose and she soon falls asleep after the oral pre-medication, holding her teddy and her mother's hand.

She is taken to theatre by her mother, Ben and the nurse, and they remain until Charlotte is anaesthetised. The nurse comforts Mrs Evans who is very anxious and offers her some tea on return to the ward. While Charlotte is in the operating theatre her bed space is prepared with a receiver, tissues and the appropriate observation charts. A check is made on the availability of oxygen and suction.

On return to the ward Charlotte is positioned correctly and her new problems are identified. Ben sits close by.

Recovery position following tonsillectomy

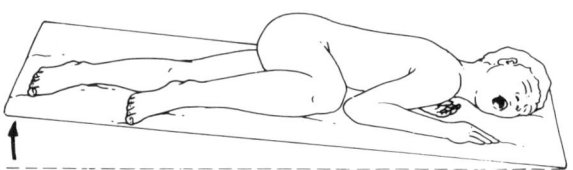

| CARE PLAN | for Charlotte postoperatively |

Potential problem: There may be bleeding from the tonsillar bed.
Nursing care and rationale: Nurse in the tonsillectomy position to maintain a clear airway and prevent inhalation of blood. Observe pulse, respiration rate, colour, excessive swallowing and restlessness to detect any reactionary haemorrhage and take action quickly if necessary. Nurse her calmly and encourage her mother to sit by her for reassurance as this may help prevent bleeding by reducing stress and anxiety.

Actual problem: She may feel pain in her throat and later otalgia (referred earache).
Nursing care and rationale: Administer prescribed analgesics, intramuscularly at first and then orally before eating to help swallowing and monitor the effects (Carrick, 1984).

Potential problem: She may be nauseated or vomit as a result of the operation.
Nursing care and rationale: Withhold all food and fluids until the likelihood of vomiting has decreased. Place receiver and tissues nearby to be prepared for vomiting, save and report all vomit, observing for blood and recording

Reactionary haemorrhage: bleeding may occur after operation and sometimes necessitates return to theatre

Nursing action:
Maintain airway by position and suction if necessary
Summon aid
Observe pulse, respiration, colour and blood loss ¼-hourly
Stay with child, comfort her and parents
Assist with preparation for theatre
Wipe blood from face and keep comfortable
Maintain intravenous infusion

volume. Gradually introduce a rough diet of the child's choice (e.g. cereal, toast) to remove slough from the fossae, starting the day after the operation. Keep her clean to preserve comfort and dignity.

Potential problem: The tonsillar bed may become infected.

Nursing care and rationale: Record temperature regularly, observe the fossae and keep the mouth clean and fresh by offering frequent oral hygiene. The method will depend on the child's age and condition.

Charlotte's father visits after work and is relieved to hear of Charlotte's progress. Her mother helps her to have a bath and go to the toilet, until she feels able to resume her independence. She is encouraged to join the other children in the play room with the play leader as soon as she feels well enough, and this gives her mother a short break and time to relax.

NURSING CARE

Evaluation

Charlotte's care is reassessed regularly; she has not developed a temperature and is eating quite well despite the soreness.

The doctor visits Charlotte and her mother and a nurse assists while he examines her. Her throat is healing well so she is told that she may go home the following day. Charlotte pronounces Ben fit too. She has received a get well card from her school class which she proudly shows around.

NURSING CARE

Planning discharge

Her father comes in to collect Charlotte and her mother and they are given the following advice to take home:

Secondary haemorrhage: this is as a result of infection and occurs around the 7th to 10th postoperative day. Signs and symptoms are pyrexia, pain and the spitting up of small amounts of blood from the fossa. Should this occur, the child is readmitted, the clot removed from the fossa and antibiotics administered.

Encourage a normal diet.

Give prescribed analgesia if required.

Return to school after a 2 week outpatient check-up.

Avoid crowded places or contact with any known infections.

Contact the G.P. if Charlotte complains of pain, fever or if there is any bleeding from her throat.

Charlotte says goodbye to all the children and nurses and her parents look relieved that her stay was less traumatic than they had expected.

Other conditions commonly found

Myringotomy and insertion of grommet. In many children, a partial deafness is caused by secretory (serous) otitis media in which there is an effusion of serous fluid in the middle ear which prevents the transmission of sound waves to the oval window.

Adenoid enlargement may also be present. This occludes the opening of the pharyngo-tympanic (Eustachian) tube. Treatment is by aspirating the fluid through a myringotomy (incision in the tympanic membrane) and usually inserting of a grommet (ventilation tube) under general anaesthesia. This equalises the pressure between the external canal and middle ear and permits the fluid to drain via the pharyngo-tympanic tube. The grommets are spontaneously extruded as the incision heals.

From the nurses point of view this child poses few specific problems apart from the deafness. Postoperatively the ear has no dressing in place and should not be touched to avoid infection. The operation may be performed as a day case or the child is discharged the following day. The parents are advised to keep the ear dry and some doctors discourage swimming for a few weeks. The main potential problem is infection of the middle ear.

Acute otitis media. This condition is also common in young children and is mostly treated at home by the G.P. As these children are rarely admitted to hospital unless they have experienced a febrile convulsion, details are not included here.

Laryngo-tracheo-bronchitis. The larynx of an infant is very small and infection may cause oedema and spasm which can be life-threatening if the child's airway becomes obstructed. Emergency admission is advised for humidification, aspiration of secretions and systemic antibiotics. If cyanosis is present an endotracheal tube may be passed and rarely a tracheostomy is performed. The problems the child experiences are dyspnoea, stridor (croup) and fear, the latter acutely felt also by the parents. The potential problems to be watched for and prevented are respiratory collapse and epiglottitis, so nursing observations are essential during the acute phase. A calm, reassuring approach from the nurse will help both the child and parent to cope with this very frightening condition. Recovery is usually fast and the child discharged quickly with the remainder of the antibiotic course and advice in case of future attacks.

TEST YOURSELF

1 What are the indications for tonsillectomy and adenoidectomy?

2 Describe the postoperative nursing care following their removal with particular reference to the complications which could occur.

3 Discuss the advice you would give parents who are unsure of how to prepare their child for admission to hospital (choose the

age of the child and relate the advice to that stage).

4 Plan the nursing care of a child readmitted to hospital with a secondary haemorrhage. What additional problems need consideration?

5 Identify the problems and plan the nursing care for a 13 month old child admitted with laryngo-tracheo-bronchitis, whose mother intends to stay in hospital with the child.

6 For some operations the child may need to be admitted for the day only. How would you prepare both parent and child and what special advice would you give as they leave the ward?

FURTHER READING

CARRICK, D. G. 1984. 'Salicylates and post-tonsillectomy haemorrhage.' *Journal of Laryngology and Otology*, **98**: 803–5.

CONSUMER'S ASSOCIATION. 1980. 'Children in Hospital.' *Which?* June.

HAMILTON SMITH, S. 1972. *Nil by Mouth? A descriptive study of nursing care in relation to preoperative fasting.* London: Royal College of Nursing.

HAWTHORN, P. 1974. *Nurse, I Want my Mummy!* London: Royal College of Nursing.

MINISTRY OF HEALTH. 1959. *The Platt Report. The Welfare of Children in Hospital.* London: HMSO.

8 The Care of the deaf

Stop for a moment and listen to all the sounds around you and try to imagine what it would be like without them or if they were distorted. This exercise may give you some insight into the feelings of the deaf, the isolation, the embarrassment at appearing stupid and being treated as such.

Hearing

Hearing is the detection of sounds by the ear and the transmission of sound impulses to the auditory centre in the brain. Deafness results when this process is disturbed, either by conductive disorders (when the mechanical conduction of sound waves to the cochlea is interrupted) or in sensori-neural deafness (when there is a defect in the cochlea or in the transmission of impulses from the cochlea to the brain).

The effects on the sufferer will vary according to the type and degree of hearing loss. A conductive loss affects all frequencies equally and the deafness is not complicated by distortion, whereas in the sensori-neural type the higher frequencies are usually affected most thus decreasing the ability to discern consonants (e.g. 's' and 't'). This renders speech incomprehensible and monotonous. To raise your voice to this person in an effort to communicate causes further distortion and distress. A conductive loss may lead the person to talk quietly because he can hear his own voice normally by bone conduction and in the absence of other sounds this appears loud so he lowers his voice to compensate. On the other hand in sensori-neural deafness all sound perception is reduced and he raises his voice in order to hear it. A person with a hearing loss may also experience other unpleasant problems, vertigo (giddiness) and tinnitus (noises in the head). Vertigo may be associated with conditions of the inner ear which affect the normal balancing function of the labyrinth. Tinnitus is an illusion of sound and is usually the result of loss of hearing and tends to be in the frequencies where the loss is most marked. It generally improves when the hearing is restored by treatment. Conductive losses are more accessible to treatment, including surgery, than sensori-neural deafness which is often helped by a hearing aid.

HISTORY

Mr and Mrs Carter arrive early for their appointment with the hearing aid technician who welcomes them and shows them into his room. The fitting and the teaching programme are carefully explained and their questions are answered, paying particular attention to slow clear speech to ensure comprehension.

An impression is taken of her outer ear from which an individual ear mould will be processed (in 2–3 weeks) and the type of aid which will best suit Mrs Carter is selected and demonstrated.

She is pleased that a 'behind the ear' aid is selected and she and her husband are taught how to use it. She is shown how to fit the mould into her ear, to replace the worn batteries, to manipulate the controls and to keep it clean. They discuss the programme of acclimatisation, beginning with an hour a day at first and gradually increasing it over a period of weeks.

She wonders why the aid is to be used in her

Hearing aids

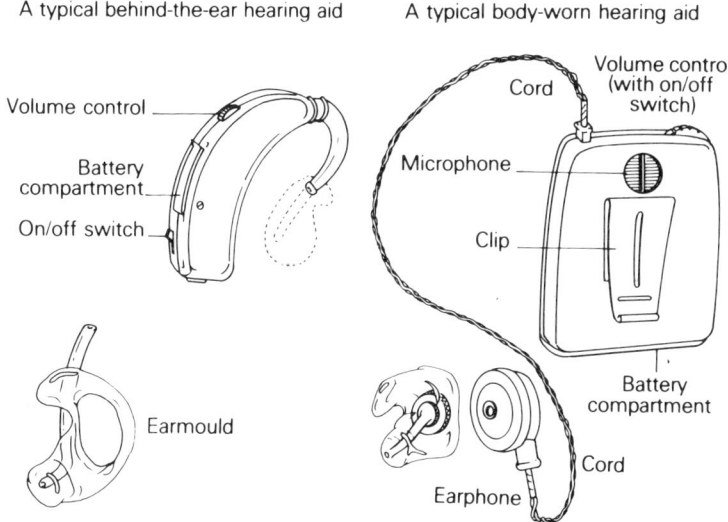

A typical behind-the-ear hearing aid

Volume control

Battery compartment

On/off switch

Earmould

A typical body-worn hearing aid

Cord

Volume control (with on/off switch)

Microphone

Clip

Battery compartment

Cord

Earphone

The post aural aid fits inconspicuously behind the ear. The controls and battery are tiny and require a degree of dexterity to manipulate them.

The body worn aid has its microphone housed in a case worn on the clothing. It may be more suitable for the very young and the very old as the controls are easier to manage.

They are both free under the National Health Service and are produced in a range of amplifications.

Switch settings: *O* means off. *N* means for normal listening. *T* means telephone – this allows the aid to pick up magnetic signals through an induction loop from the telephone or television. This system amplifies the voice only and excludes background noise. Many churches, theatres and cinemas have a loop system installed. Emergency telephones on motorways are also fitted with this facility.

M allows the listener to hear through the hearing aid microphone.

MT permits use of the microphone and induction loop simultaneously.

H means low tones are filtered out which may help reduce background noise.

right (better hearing) ear and the technician explains that in her case the quality of hearing will be better.

They are told that a hearing aid simply amplifies sound, that it does not select or interpret; therefore all sounds will be louder, including the background ones which are normally filtered out and ignored. Also a hearing aid is most effective when the speaker is about 7 feet away (something for the nurse to remember when speaking to a patient). Mr and Mrs Carter are asked to think about what they want from the hearing aid and this information will form the basis of a contract for use and enable them to evaluate its success in terms of how much it has fulfilled their need. They leave with this task in mind, to return for the hearing aid when the mould is ready.

When they return Mrs Carter is again shown how to fit the aid correctly and she practises with the help of the technician. They discuss the aspects about which she is unsure and Mr and Mrs Carter leave with high hopes of what help it will bring them. After a few weeks of increasing use she visits the department to discuss her progress and is introduced to the hearing therapist who will continue her care.

Hearing therapy: 'The role of the Hearing Therapist is that of educating hard of hearing adults, their families and associates, to facilitate a return to as normal a communication style as is possible within the limits of their hearing impairment. This includes an aural rehabilitation programme, the aim of which is to revive their memory of sounds, and to teach them to recognise the sounds they now hear as having the same meaning as the sounds they remember before acquiring their hearing loss' (Levene, 1984).

The programme also includes lipreading, help with the hearing aid and advice about environmental aids (such as an amplified handset for the telephone). If the person needs aids to assist him in his work these may be acquired through the Disablement Resettlement Officer. Hearing therapy is a recent innovation in the care of the hearing impaired and it may be some years before every department has a therapist.

A tailor-made programme of weekly sessions is planned for Mrs Carter during which the above aspects will be covered. Positive reinforcement and encouragement are essential aspects of the approach by the hearing therapist (success depends on the development of a supportive, relaxed relationship within which both parties can function).

After the first of these sessions Mr and Mrs Carter feel confident that at the end of the programme her difficulties in communication will be greatly improved.

Advice for nurses when communicating with the hearing impaired (from Levene, 1983)

Be patient
Attract the person's attention before speaking by touch or moving to where you can be seen
Sit with the light on your face
Sit on the same level as the person
Look at the person when speaking
Do not speak with your face covered, avoid mannerisms that temporarily hide your lips and keep your hands still
Do not shout
Speak slowly and distinctly in a moderate voice
Do not exaggerate lip movements
Write down important facts
Ensure that the person's glasses are clean
Check the hearing aid is working
If in a group avoid asides to others in the group
Take the person to a quiet area in the ward/ department if there is a lot of extraneous noise

Hearing aids – Fault finding chart
'Behind the ear' hearing aids

Symptoms	Fault	Action
Aid dead	Earmould blocked with wax Battery reversed or flat Contacts dirty	Remove earmold and clean Examine, test and replace
Rushing noise from aid	Switch in T position Microphone not working	Reset switch to M position Return aid for repair
Low output from aid	Wrong setting of output/tone control Mould or tubing blocked Tubing kinked	Reset controls Return aid for repair Remove blockage Replace tube
Crackling	Faulty connections	Clean contacts if possible
Acoustic Feedback	Poorly fitting earmould Tubing split	Check fit of earmould Renew Replace tube

Bodyworn hearing aids

When testing aid, keep earphone and microphone 30–45 cm apart. Turn right up; if there still is no sound, aid is faulty.

Aid dead	Earmould blocked with wax Battery reversed or flat Contacts dirty or broken Cord broken Faulty receiver or socket Faulty socket	Unclip from receiver and clean Examine and replace Wiggle cord near plugs Renew Replace Move cord in and out of socket Return aid for repair
Rushing noise from aid	Switch in T position Microphone not working	Switch to M position Return aid for repair

Low output from aid	Low voltage battery	Change battery
	Faulty or wrong receiver	Replace
	Wrong setting of output/tone control	Reset controls
Crackling	Damaged cord, dirty volume control	Replace cord Clean volume control
	Faulty socket	Return aid
Acoustic feedback	Poorly fitting earmould	Check fit of earmould Renew
Stuttering sound	Low voltage causing electrical instability	Change battery
		Clean contacts

(Adapted from the original by M C Martin of the Royal National Institute for the Deaf, London.)

TEST YOURSELF

1 How would you teach a junior nurse to communicate with a hard of hearing patient?

2 In what ways may the home life of a deafened person be improved?

3 Discuss ways in which you may help a patient who is deaf to cope when admitted for an unrelated condition to a general ward. One example might be to encourage the wearing of his hearing aid to the anaesthetic room, to aid communication.

4 What do you feel are the wider implications of hearing loss to an individual?

FURTHER READING

LEVENE, B. 1983. 'Hearing Loss – the Invisible Disability'. *Nursing*, 2, No 18.
LEVENE, B. 1984. The Role of the Hearing Therapist (unpublished notes).

9 Nursing Mrs Scott who is undergoing ear surgery

You will encounter a variety of ear conditions, some requiring operation, during your experience in the ear, nose and throat ward. One such case history is discussed here in detail and this may be used as a framework for planning the care of the other patients you meet. Two others are briefly mentioned at the end of the chapter.

HISTORY

Mrs Scott is a 43 year old housewife with no children. She has experienced increasing deafness in both ears over the past few years and was referred to the Ear, Nose and Throat outpatients by her G.P. After investigation, the diagnosis of otosclerosis was made and an operation, stapedectomy, was offered for her poorer hearing ear (right). Her interests include reading, knitting and watching television. She neither smokes nor drinks alcohol.

Mrs Scott is admitted accompanied by her husband; they are both welcomed and shown to her bed. Mrs Scott has considerable difficulty in hearing normal conversation so great care is taken by the nurse to face her when talking to her, speaking slowly, clearly and at the normal volume, making sure she has understood completely. She is very nervous, mainly, she says, because of the deafness and the fear of missing information and appearing to be stupid. When she has unpacked her case

Otosclerosis: otosclerosis causes deafness by fixing or immobilising the stapes in the oval window with an overgrowth of bone. It is usually bilateral but at different stages in the two ears. It is more common in women, is familial and may begin during pregnancy. It causes a conductive hearing loss demonstrated by this audiogram.

Audiogram showing conductive deafness

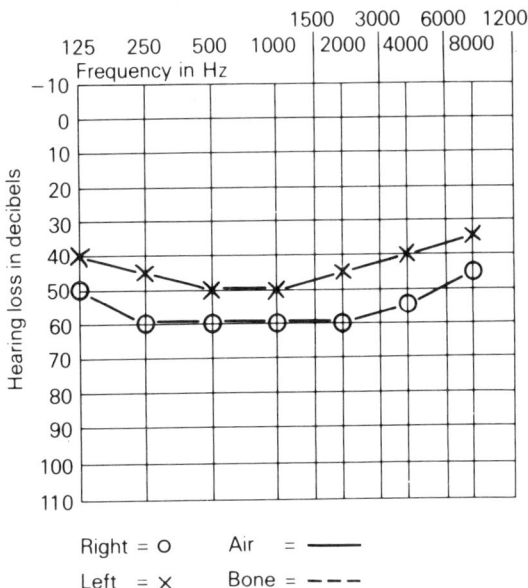

Right = O   Air = ——

Left = ✕   Bone = — — —

Treatment may be by prescribing a hearing aid or by the operation stapedectomy.

The middle ear is entered by turning back the intact tympanic membrane, removing the stapes in whole or part, replacing it with a prosthesis and restoring the tympanic membrane.

teflon prosthesis

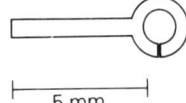

5 mm

The operation, using an operating microscope, is highly successful but does carry the possibility of serious complications e.g. complete sensori-neural deafness and failure of the labyrinth ('dead ear'), of which the patient should be warned.

she and her husband are shown around the ward and the ward routine is carefully explained to her. A nursing history is taken and the doctor visits to examine Mrs Scott and discuss the proposed operation with them both. The unlikely complication of 'dead ear' is explained and Mrs Scott signs a consent form. He marks her right ear to ensure the correct one is treated.

From the information gained, the nurse together with Mrs Scott plans the pre-operative care.

| CARE PLAN | for Mrs Scott pre-operatively |

Actual problem: She is very deaf from the otosclerosis.
Nursing care and rationale: Spend time in communication and use a paper and pencil for important details if necessary.

Actual problem: She is frightened because of her isolation and the proposed operation.
Nursing care and rationale: Offer full explanations of treatment and nursing care. To reduce her feeling of isolation ensure that all staff and relevant other patients are aware of her difficulties.

Potential problem: Postoperative coughing may dislodge the prosthesis.
Nursing care and rationale: Teach her breathing exercises and ensure that the lung fields are clear pre-operatively to help prevent coughing.

Mrs Scott's preparation continues by explaining in detail her nursing care postoperatively as co-operation will increase the likelihood of success. She feels more settled now that she understands all that is involved. She washes her hair to reduce the possibility of infection.

The nurse who accompanies Mrs Scott to

theatre remains until she is anaesthetised to reassure her and ensure that the theatre staff are aware of her hearing difficulty.

On return from the operation Mrs Scott's specific problems are identified by the nurse and her nursing aims are established.

CARE PLAN

for Mrs Scott postoperatively

Potential problem: She may suffer from vertigo as a result of disturbing the oval window, leading to nausea and vomiting.

Nursing care and rationale: Nurse flat with one pillow on the unaffected side and avoid sudden head movements (including sneezing, coughing or vomiting) to prevent perilymph leaking before the entrance is sealed and dislodging of the prosthesis. When no vertigo is present, sit her up gradually and encourage her to resume activities as she feels capable. Administer regular anti-emetics as prescribed (which also serve as labyrinthine suppressant).

Actual problem: She will be more deaf as a result of the dressing in her ear and lying on her better hearing ear.

Nursing care and rationale: Approach her carefully and speak clearly to avoid startling her. Place a bell or buzzer within reach at all times so that she can summon help. Observe the dressing at regular intervals for bleeding or discharge but leave untouched. Monitor her temperature four hourly to detect the development of infection.

Actual problem: She is lying flat on her side in bed.

Nursing care and rationale: Offer toilet facilities regularly, and sit her up carefully on a commode if she is unable to eliminate lying flat. To maintain diet and hydration provide her meals in such a way that they can be consumed horizontally.

If the patient experiences vertigo (characterised by the presence of nystagmus) at any stage in the mobilisation programme she should return to the position which did not cause it and the programme delayed until improvement occurs.

61

Mr Scott visits frequently, bearing bunches of flowers he has grown himself. He is very relieved when he sees his wife getting up and about although she is still a little unsure of her balance at times.

Evaluation

Regular reassessment of her nursing aims reveals no complications and she is coping well in the strange environment despite her hearing difficulties.

After four days she feels more confident, is no longer giddy, is eating well and thinks her hearing has improved. This is proved when her external auditory canal dressing is removed before she is discharged.

Planning discharge

Mr Scott is taking a week's holiday so he can look after her when she goes home. She is advised to avoid loud, noisy places at first as these may be unpleasant, having suddenly recaptured some hearing; instead she should gradually expose herself to build up her tolerance. Other advice is discussed:

Avoid situations which alter the middle ear pressure (e.g. flying and high buildings). Resist nose blowing as this may introduce infection via the pharyngo-tympanic tube. Keep the ear dry and avoid interference.

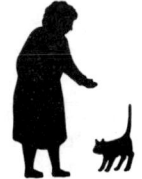

She is given an outpatient appointment for one month when an audiogram will be done to record her hearing improvement. As Mr and Mrs Scott leave she says she is looking forward to hearing her cat purr for the first time.

Other conditions commonly found

Myringoplasty. A perforation of the tympanic membrane will cause conductive deafness. It may be the result of acute otitis media or injury but in order to close the middle ear and restore the hearing, myringoplasty is performed. The defect is closed with a graft (e.g. of temporal fascia) and kept in position by a dressing (BIPP) in the external auditory canal which may be left in place for 2–3 weeks to allow the graft to take.

The patient presents similar problems to those covered above, but as vertigo is unlikely mobilisation occurs earlier. The donor site is shaved pre-operatively and its sutures removed when healed. Similar advice is offered to the patient on discharge, particularly stressing the avoidance of sneezing with a closed mouth and nose blowing as both these activities may disturb the graft.

Chronic suppurative otitis media. This condition, characterised by purulent discharge from the ear and deafness, is often associated with cholesteatoma formation (a collection of epithelial debris) in the roof of the middle ear, which increases in size eroding the surrounding structures which may include the ossicles, mastoid air cells and facial nerve. As a result of its invasive nature and the possibility of intracranial complications the ear is 'made safe' either by regular local suction or operation. A variety of operations are performed with the combined aim of safety and preservation of remaining hearing, e.g. mastoidectomy and tympanoplasty. The patient returns from the operation with a wound either in front or behind the pinna and a cavity dressing of BIPP. Postoperatively frequent observations of facial symmetry are carried out to detect damage to or compression of the facial nerve.

The dressing is removed when the cavity has

healed and the patient is asked to return frequently for checks to detect regrowth of the cholesteatoma.

1 What is otosclerosis and why does it result in deafness?

2 Construct a nursing care plan for a patient during the first 48 hours following stapedectomy.

3 What are the complications of middle ear disease and how would you recognise them?

4 In the unlikely event of 'death' of the labyrinth following stapedectomy, how would you help the patient come to terms with the tragedy and plan for her future?

10 Nursing Mr Sanchez with a tracheostomy

HISTORY

Mr Luis Sanchez is a 60 year old Spaniard who although resident in England for twenty years speaks little English. He is admitted, accompanied by his wife, as a planned admission for surgical removal of carcinoma of his tongue. He has had a painful ulcer on his tongue for three months and it has been investigated in the outpatient department and admission advised following the biopsy result. They have no children and Mr Sanchez is retired but his wife works as a domestic in the hospital. He smokes a pipe, drinks socially and is rather underweight because eating is very painful.

During the operation and for a few days afterwards Mr Sanchez will have a temporary tracheostomy in order to reduce the threat to his airway by tongue and pharyngeal swelling.

Tracheostomy: a tracheostomy is an artificial opening in the trachea into which a tube is inserted. Air enters via the stoma, bypassing the normal filtering, moistening and warming functions performed by the nasal mucosa. As a result the trachea is more susceptible to drying and infection.

Indications for tracheostomy:

Obstruction of upper respiratory tract from:	Oedema, burns
	Foreign body
	Laryngeal injury, paralysis
	Laryngo-tracheo-bronchitis
	Laryngeal carcinoma
Protection of bronchial tree from aspiration in:	Bulbar poliomyelitis
	Myasthenia gravis
	Coma
Cleaning of bronchial tree in:	Pulmonary disease (e.g. pneumonia)
	Suppression of cough reflex

Ventilation	Disorders of respiratory centre
to provide	'Flail' chest
long-term	Disorders of respiratory muscles
intermittent	
positive pressure	
ventilation in:	

Tracheostomy may be performed for more than one of these reasons on the same patient.

Initial stages

Mr and Mrs Sanchez are welcomed and shown to his room. He appears fairly cheerful but Mrs Sanchez is anxious. She speaks better English than her husband, but to ensure complete comprehension a Spanish interpreter is found and all communications are conducted through him. When he is settled and unpacked a nurse shows them around the ward and takes a nursing history.

The doctor visits and in the presence of the interpreter carefully explains what the treatment and care will entail.

Mrs Sanchez asks many questions particularly related to the temporary tracheostomy which seems to cause them both more anxiety than the operation or the presence of cancer itself. (From here the care discussed will relate to the tracheostomy only.)

Tracheostomy in position

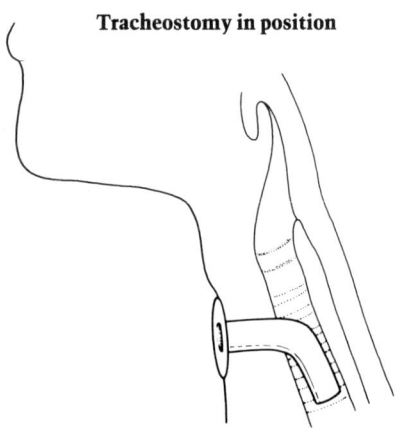

The incision is made in front of the trachea between the 2nd and 3rd or 3rd and 4th cartilagenous tracheal rings.

Skin sutures may be necessary. The largest tracheostomy tube which will fit comfortably is inserted and the cuff, which is situated at the lower end, inflated until an airtight seal is achieved. The wound may be dressed with a non-adherent dressing and the tube tapes securely fastened at the neck. As long as the larynx remains, speech is possible by deflating the cuff and covering the stoma thus redirecting expired air through the larynx and mouth. This assumes there is enough space between the tube and the tracheal wall, i.e. the cuff must be deflated.

From the nursing history the nurse identifies Mr Sanchez's pre-operative problems and together they plan his care, again using the interpreter.

CARE PLAN

for Mr Sanchez pre-operatively

Actual problem: He is very anxious about the proposed operation especially as his English is so limited.

Nursing care and rationale: Offer full explanations of all that is happening through a Spanish interpreter. Find out about any social problems and deal with them appropriately, keeping him informed of the results. Establish a reliable method of communication to be used after surgery, including language cards or photographic communication charts if necessary.

Actual problem: He regularly smokes a pipe which may increase the risk of chest complications.

Nursing care and rationale: Tactfully explain the risks of pipe smoking through the interpreter and help him to find ways of giving up. Teach breathing exercises to help prevent chest complications. (It may be kinder not to identify the connection between smoking and carcinoma at this stage.)

Actual problem: He is underweight and thus possibly malnourished and weak.

Nursing care and rationale: Offer him an appetising diet and extra nutritious drinks to increase weight and improve his general health. Ask his wife to bring in his favourite food, particularly as the hospital food may be very different from the food he eats at home. This also involves his wife actively in his care thus lessening her anxiety.

During the few days prior to the operation, frequent discussions occur to clarify the information. With the help of the interpreter all aspects of the tracheostomy are covered, slowly and patiently, the site of the stoma, the nursing care and the equipment that will be required to carry it out. A reliable method of communication is established and they are told that one nurse will be with him constantly for the first day or two. His temporary loss of speech causes him some anxiety but it helps when he hears that his wife may visit him at any time.

One of the nurses on the ward speaks some Spanish so it is planned that she should look after him as much as possible. She prepares him for operation and takes him to the operating theatre.

While Mr Sanchez is in the operating theatre his room is prepared to receive him.

As Mr Sanchez returns to the ward his new problems are identified, the nursing aims are established and his care is planned.

| CARE PLAN | for Mr Sanchez postoperatively |

Actual problem: He has a tracheostomy which must be maintained clear.

Nursing care and rationale: Observe respiratory rate and freedom, skin colour, pulse and

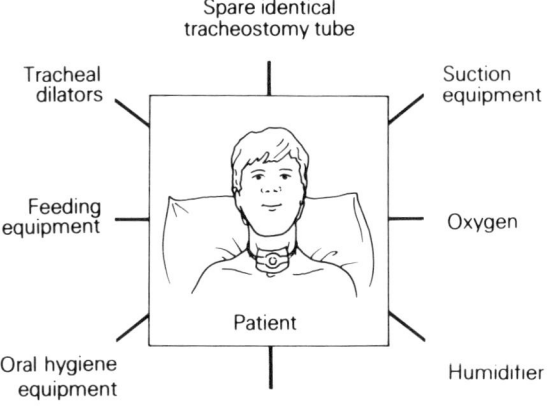

Spare identical
tracheostomy tube

Tracheal
dilators

Suction
equipment

Feeding
equipment

Oxygen

Oral hygiene
equipment

Humidifier

Patient

Means of communication:
bell or buzzer,
paper and pencil

blood pressure to monitor his condition. Nurse him sitting upright (when his condition allows) well supported by pillows to aid chest expansion. Aspirate the tracheostomy quarter hourly at first, gradually reducing the frequency as the secretions diminish. Encourage breathing exercises at frequent intervals. Administer humidified air (or oxygen if prescribed) continuously, first through a blower humidifier and then progressing to a specially designed bib (e.g. Buchanan bib). This filters

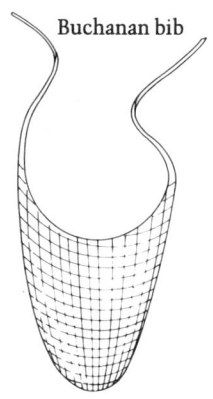

Buchanan bib

the inspired air and gives it the warmth and humidity it would normally receive from going through the mouth or nose and prevents crusting of the mucous membrane. Change the tracheostomy tube daily (after the first change by the surgeon 48 hours after the operation), progressing to a silver tube as indicated. Replace dressings and tapes as necessary, observing the stoma for signs of bleeding and infection. Maintain the inflation of the tube cuff until wound oozing has ceased and then progress to an uncuffed tube. This helps to prevent inspiration pneumonia. To maintain hydration and nutrition, offer a normal diet if he is conscious and the swallowing reflex is present; otherwise give a liquidised diet through a nasogastric tube.

Actual problem: He is unable to speak.

Nursing care: Watch for signs of withdrawal or depression due to this and give reassurance to increase his confidence and lessen fear. Ensure a bell or buzzer and paper and pencil are nearby at all times. Remain with him for the first 24–48 hours so any airway problems can be dealt with promptly.

Tracheal aspiration: This is an aseptic procedure so gloves and a new sterile catheter are used for each aspiration. The suction equipment is changed and sterilised daily.

The size of the catheter should be less than half the tracheostomy tube diameter to prevent hypoxia and to reduce the negative pressure being exerted on the lungs.

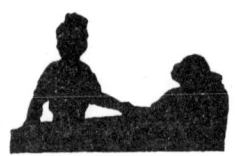

The suction pressure required is 150–200cm water; if higher the catheter may adhere to the tracheal mucosa and cause damage.

Suction should only be applied during withdrawal of the catheter, so it is either compressed on introduction or a Y-connection is used.

The frequency of aspiration varies widely according to the volume of secretions but during the first 24 hours aspiration should be performed quarter to half hourly. In the drowsy postoperative phase secretions will collect and the irritation that leads to coughing will be reduced.

Regular, planned aspiration should be performed, not left to 'whenever necessary'.

The catheter is inserted deep enough into the trachea to stimulate coughing; deeper insertion is rarely indicated and causes unnecessary discomfort.

To prevent hypoxia, suction should not be applied for longer than 10–15 seconds without a significant rest.

Frequent inexperienced reinflation of the cuff may be more dangerous than once daily deflation when the tube is changed. Over inflation causes tracheal ischaemia and necrosis. For this reason the smallest volume of air is injected that achieves a seal, and no air can be heard escaping. The use of a cuff pressure gauge will avoid the dangers of over- or under-inflation.

Mrs Sanchez visits frequently during the day and in the evening. She begins to look more relaxed as she sees her husband's progress. As he is out of bed, coping well with his diet and his mouth swelling has decreased, the doctors are planning to remove his tracheostomy tube to enable him to breathe normally again. Mr and Mrs Sanchez are very pleased by this decision and the method of closure is fully explained to them both with the help of the interpreter.

The tracheostomy tube is blocked off with a sterile cork or tape for 24 hours and Mr Sanchez is carefully observed for signs of difficulty with breathing especially during the night when asleep. He manages well and is very pleased that he is able to speak again albeit indistinctly (because of the tongue surgery). With patience he can be understood.

The following day the tube is removed and the opening is sealed off with an airtight dressing. After a few more days the wound has closed over and he is breathing normally through his mouth and nose.

Occasionally when the stoma has been established for a long period closure by suturing is necessary.

He is encouraged to continue his breathing exercises and any sputum is expectorated via his mouth. He has wisely decided to give up pipe smoking, much to his wife's relief.

Diagram of tubes

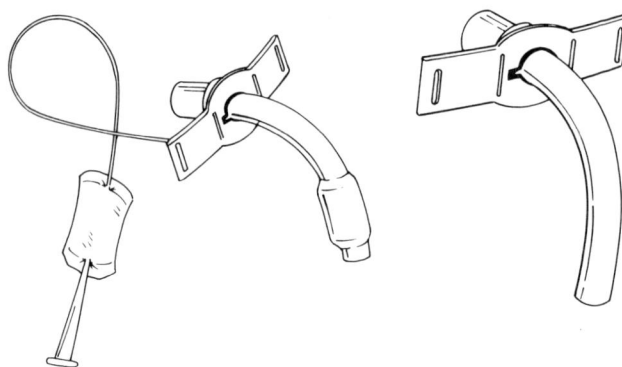

Portex standard cuff
tracheostomy tube

Portex plain
tracheostomy tube

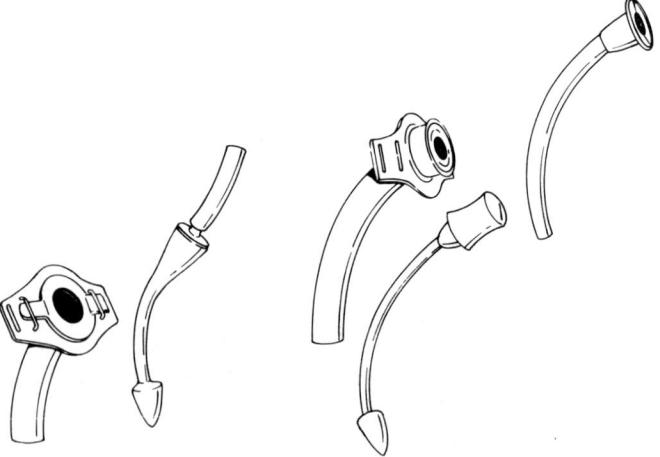

Colledge laryngectomy
tube with introducer

Negus tracheostomy tube
with introducer and inner
tubes (one plain and one
with 'speaking' valve)

Changing of tracheostomy tube

1. Aspirate the tracheostomy,

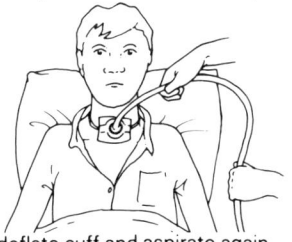 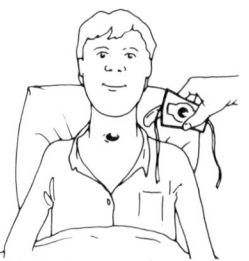

deflate cuff and aspirate again
(to remove secretions which
had collected above the cuff).

2. Untie tapes and remove
tube and dressing

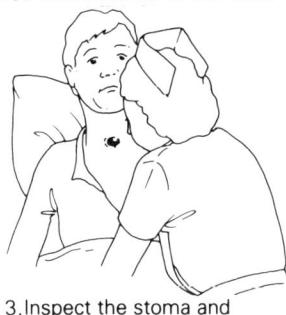 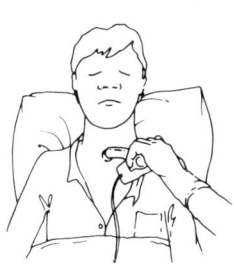

3. Inspect the stoma and
clean if necessary

4. Insert sterile tube

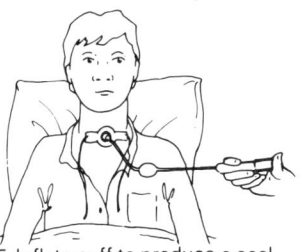 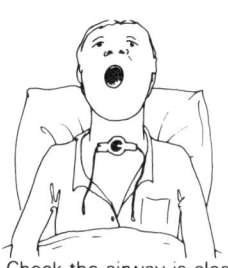

5. Inflate cuff to produce a seal

6. Check the airway is clear

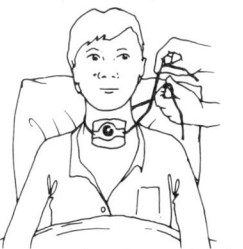 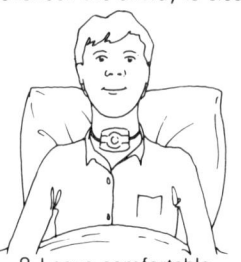

7. Place dressing under the
tube and tie tapes

8. Leave comfortable

Evaluation

At each stage of his progress evaluation is carried out and any required changes in his care made. He developed none of the potential problems.

Mr Sanchez is making good progress and from the tracheostomy point of view no further intervention is indicated. The remainder of his time in hospital is involved with rehabilitating him with regard to his mouth, eating and speech.

1 What are the indications for tracheostomy?

2 How would you prepare a patient for a temporary tracheostomy?

3 Construct a nursing care plan using the problem solving approach, for his care in the first 48 hours after surgery.

4 How would you ensure good communications continued during that time?

5 For certain conditions (e.g. paralysis of the vocal cords) permanent tracheostomy may be indicated. Discuss the reasons for this and how your nursing care might be affected.

Nursing Mr Green who is undergoing a Laryngectomy

Mr William Green is a 55 year old garage mechanic who was widowed a year ago and has two married daughters. He lives in a council house on his own and looks after himself with help from his daughters who live nearby. His interests are gardening, his four grandchildren, aged between 4 and 10 years, and meeting his friends in the local public house to play darts once a week. He drinks socially and smokes 30 cigarettes a day.

Mr Green has been hoarse for six months and his daughters have persuaded him to see his doctor, who has referred him to the ENT Clinic urgently, suspecting a carcinoma of the vocal cords, and admission is arranged to investigate his symptoms under general anaesthetic.

Carcinoma of the larynx: carcinoma of the larynx accounts for 2% of the UK total malignancies. It may arise in the vocal cords, causing hoarseness, or above or below them, causing respiratory distress, dysphagia, pain, bleeding or metastases. Tumours which arise on the vocal cord and are diagnosed early may often be cured by radiotherapy. Most laryngeal carcinomas are squamous cell in origin and the degree of cell differentiation determines the speed of growth (e.g. poorly differentiated tumours grow rapidly and tend to metastasise more readily).

Initial stages

Mr Green and his daughters are welcomed and shown to his bed. He is very anxious, having considered the possibility of cancer. After his

Direct laryngoscopy: direct laryngoscopy enables the surgeon to see the interior of the larynx, to assess the presence, position and extent of the tumour and to take a biopsy for histological investigation.

daughters have helped him unpack a nurse shows them around the ward and takes a nursing history. He asks for his daughters to stay to help him answer the questions. Following the doctor's examination, his treatment is discussed with his daughters present. They are told that a small investigation under an anaesthetic will reveal the cause of his hoarseness. He asks how long it will be before the result is confirmed. This and their other questions are answered carefully. The nurse then involves Mr Green in planning his care for the operation the following day.

| CARE PLAN | for Mr Green pre-operatively |

Actual problem: Anxiety caused by the uncertainty of the diagnosis and hospital admission.
Nursing care: Offer full explanations of the nursing care and treatment. Deal with any social problems he may have.

Actual problem: Cigarette smoking.
Nursing care: Tactfully explain to him the hazards of continuing cigarette smoking and find ways to help him give up.

Mr Green is prepared and accompanied to the operating theatre. On his return to the ward his new problems are identified by the nurse and his care planned accordingly.

| CARE PLAN | for Mr Green postoperatively |

Potential problem: The airway may become obstructed by tongue, vomit or as a result of laryngeal swelling and oozing.
Nursing care and rationale: Nurse in a flat lateral position until fully awake and observe respiratory rate and freedom and skin colour

Generally carcinoma of the larynx is treated by radiotherapy. If radiotherapy fails or the tumour is unsuitable for it, a laryngectomy will be performed.

for signs of respiratory difficulties. Check that the cough reflex has returned before offering him fluids, as a local laryngeal anaesthetic may be used in conjunction with the general anaesthetic. Encourage deep breathing exercises when he is awake to help prevent chest infection.

Mr Green's anxiety remains and the nurses talk to him at length to support him whilst awaiting the biopsy report. The histology report confirms the diagnosis of carcinoma.

Mr Green and his daughters are told of the diagnosis by the Consultant and that the treatment of choice is laryngectomy. They talk over the details and the doctor promises to return to answer further questions they may have. The nurse follows this with more in-

The neck before and after laryngectomy

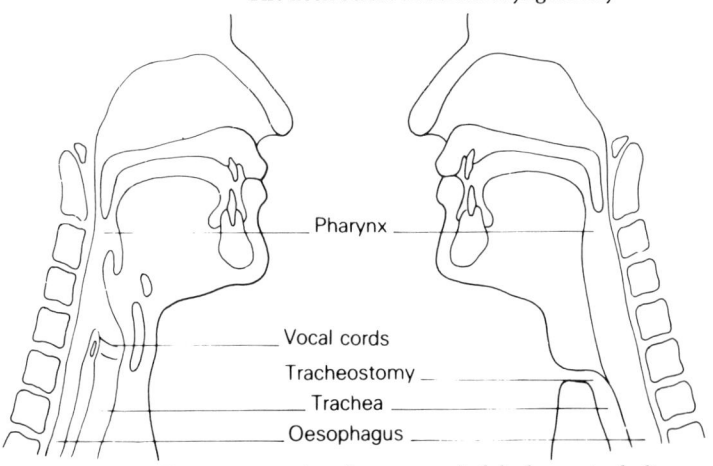

Laryngectomy involves removal of the larynx including the epiglottis, hyoid bone, thyroid and cricoid cartilages and 2 or 3 tracheal rings. The pharyngeal wall is closed and temporary nasogastric feeding commenced. The opening of the trachea is sutured to the skin to form a permanent tracheostomy. The neck wound is drained by using two vacuum type drainage tubes. It is sometimes also necessary to remove affected lymph nodes by block dissection.

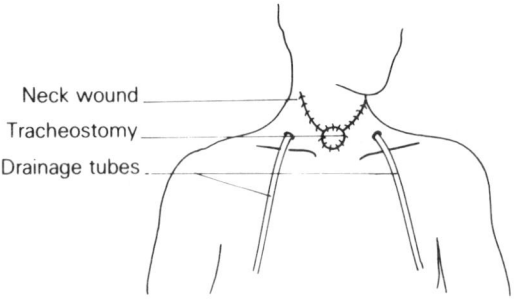

Diagram of neck wound

Neck wound
Tracheostomy
Drainage tubes

formation concerning the removal of his normal method of speech and the creation of a stoma in his neck and explains what all this will mean to him and his family. He says that he thought he might need this operation and although it is a shock, he feels more settled now the uncertainty has passed.

Mr Green is slowly and carefully prepared for laryngectomy ensuring that he and his family understand all that is involved (Start, 1985).

He is visited by various people who will be closely involved in his care and rehabilitation. One of his daughters arranges to be with him when any of the following visit to help him grasp the details.

Physiotherapist: explains exercises and tracheal aspiration

Medical Social Worker: visits to help solve any social problems and assess the suitability of his job for his return

Speech Therapist: discusses the new type of speech he will be taught and helps establish a temporary method for the interim (Is he literate? as pencil and paper are often used)

Another patient: visits to describe his experiences, demonstrate oesophageal speech and answer any questions.

His pre-operative care is similar to that given before but more time is devoted to explaining the nursing care, the equipment to be used in his care, the wound and 'tubes' which will be in use, and what means he will use to communicate immediately after surgery (Hayward, 1975). A nurse accompanies him to the operating theatre and while he is there his room is prepared (see p. 69).

A familiar nurse collects him from the operation and identifies his new problems, establishes his nursing aims and plans his subsequent care.

The following care plan relates specifically to his care following removal of his larynx, and not to the tracheostomy (p. 68).

<table>
<tr><td>

CARE PLAN

</td><td>

for Mr Green postoperatively

</td></tr>
</table>

Actual problem: He has had his larynx removed and an end tracheostomy fashioned.

Nursing care and rationale: Observe neck wounds for bleeding and any signs of infection. Maintain the drainage tubes to prevent haematoma formation under the flap, changing them as required and remove them when drainage ceases. If there is any pain, administer the prescribed analgesic as necessary and monitor the effect. Feed him a liquidised diet through a nasogastric tube until the pharyngeal repair has healed to prevent leakage. Offer sterile fluids, progressing to a normal diet when it is tolerated. Remove sutures when wound is healed.

The pharyngeal repair is tested by swallowing radio-opaque fluid. If leakage is demonstrated on X-ray, fluids are withheld until the fistula (track between pharynx and stoma) has closed.

Actual problem: He is unable to speak.
Nursing care and rationale: To prevent frustra-

tion because of his voice loss, take time to understand his needs and ensure that there is some means of communication at hand. Encourage practice of speech therapy exercises when indicated.

Oesophageal speech: oesophageal speech may be taught as soon as the patient is eating normally. It involves injection of air into the top of the oesophagus and then its expulsion which vibrates to produce voice at the pharyngo-oesophageal junction. About 33% of patients following laryngectomy achieve good oesophageal voices. Other options are the artificial larynx of the intra oral or neck type (they generate sound electronically which is articulated by the patient) or the surgically constructed tracheo-oesophageal fistula and valve insertion.

Mr Green becomes mobile very quickly and his neck feels more comfortable too. His daughters and their children visit him regularly and this helps to keep him cheerful, the children appear unaffected by his tube, just pleased to see their grandfather well. The nurses and doctors talk to Mr Green and his family at regular intervals to discuss his progress and plan for the future.

NURSING CARE

Evaluation

Regular evaluation of his care is carried out and intervention is altered accordingly, he is not developing any specific complications, e.g. chest or wound infection, tracheo-pharyngeal fistula or depression, and is communicating well.

NURSING CARE

Rehabilitation

Throughout his stay Mr Green's care has been aimed at rehabilitation and discharge home. He is gradually introduced to his tracheostomy and its care, including tube changing, cleaning and suction, using a mirror to view it. These procedures are taught in a relaxed unhurried atmosphere to build up his confidence and reduce his anxiety and squeamishness. (Occasionally a relative may need to perform them for the patient.)

He is given the following equipment to take home, and told where he may obtain replacements:

Portable suction apparatus
Sterile catheters
2 laryngectomy tubes and introducers
Tape for the tube
Cleaning equipment for the tube
Stoma bibs

Before he goes home, speech therapy and outpatient appointments are arranged and the patient who has visited him throughout his stay introduces him to the local club for laryngectomy patients. Mr Green finds this useful and it encourages him to persevere with his oesophageal speech exercises. He is reminded of the potential problems he may face, e.g. the dangers of water in the stoma and of dry smoky atmospheres. He had noticed that his sense of smell had been reduced because he could not now sniff or blow his nose. He is encouraged to dress as normally as possible, and will soon become used to the feeling of light clothing covering his stoma. He is advised to carry a card stating that in an emergency resuscitation must be applied to his stoma and this reassures him.

The garage has been very helpful and is expecting him back after two months convalescence at home. As he does not need to talk for long periods when at work his return poses no problems.

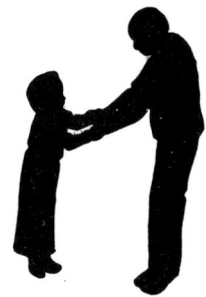

When he is completely confident about looking after himself, he arranges to go home and one of his daughters decides to stay with him for a few days to ensure that he is able to cope. Mr Green thinks his grandchildren are likely to encourage him to practice his oesophageal voice more than anyone else.

1 What are the problems a patient with cancer of the larynx may encounter?

2 What methods are used to diagnose the condition?

3 How would you prepare a patient for laryngectomy?

4 Construct a nursing care plan for his postoperative period.

5 How would you teach a patient to aspirate his tracheostomy himself?

6 What preparations will need to be made to enable a patient to go home after laryngectomy?

7 What advice do you feel would help him to adjust to his normal life style?

8 Many patients are treated with radiotherapy with or without chemotherapy; consider the special needs and care involved whilst the patient is receiving these treatments.

9 For hypopharyngeal tumours pharyngo-laryngo-oesophagectomy is indicated. This will require an oesophageal replacement using the stomach or small intestine. What additional problems will this patient present and how will the nurse solve them?

FURTHER
READING

HAYWARD, J. 1975. *Information – A Prescription against Pain*. London: Royal College of Nursing.
START, K. M. 1985. 'Assessment of patient and nurse experiences in pre-operative teaching of laryngectomy patients.' To be completed as part of BSc (Hons) Nursing Studies. NESCOT.

12 Conclusion

If the author has succeeded in interesting you in ear, nose and throat nursing, you may now wish to increase your knowledge of this specialty by reading the recommended books. You may also like to read the reports of related research which may be found in documents or journals. New findings which affect nursing care are frequently being reported and it is important for nurses to keep up-to-date and use research findings in their care.

As you will know, patients who are deaf or have speech difficulties are frequently encountered in general medical and surgical wards and units for the elderly. You will find the skills in communication that you have learnt from your experience in the Ear, Nose and Throat Unit invaluable. You will also have the information to hand to investigate a patient's malfunctioning hearing aid and help to restore the aid to normal, instead of replacing it in the locker.

USEFUL ADDRESSES

Association of Teachers of Lip
Reading for Adults
Miss J. Wilson, Information
Officer
c/o Slimbridge Post Office
Gloucestershire

British Association of the Hard of
Hearing
7–11 Armstrong Road
London w3
01-743–1110

Disablement Rehabilitation
Officer
Main Job Centres

National Association of
Laryngectomee Clubs
4th floor
39 Eccleston Square
London swiv ipb
01-834–2857

National Association for the
Welfare of Children in Hospital
Argyl House
29–31 Euston Road
London nwi 2sd
01-833–2041

Photographic Teaching Materials
23 Horn Street
Winslow
Bucks

Royal National Institute for the
Deaf
105 Gower Street
London wci
01-387–8033

INDEX

Fungus 20

Gastrointestinal
tract 13
Glomerulonephritis
44
Graft 63
Grommet (ventilation
tube) 48

Haematoma 79
Haemoglobin 8, 23,
24, 26
Haemolytic
streptococcus 44
Haemorrhage 39, 40,
46–8, 50, 61, 69, 75,
79
Halitosis 29
Headache, frontal 32,
34
Health Visitor 43
Hearing 51, 62, 63
air conduction 18
bone conduction 18
Hearing aids 18, 52–7,
59, 83
Hearing tests 17
tuning fork 18, 22
Hearing therapy 54,
55
Hereditary
telangiectasia 23
Hoarseness 75, 76
Humidification 49, 69
Hypertension 23, 26
Hypoxia 70, 71

Infection 2, 40
intravenous infusion
site 30, 34
middle ear 18, 43,
49, 61
respiratory tract 24,
65, 76, 80
sinus 32, 34, 36
tonsil 47
upper respiratory
tract 28
wound 35, 48, 60,
70, 79, 80
Inflammation 30
Insomnia 39
Itching 20, 21

Labyrinth 52, 59, 64
suppressant 61
Laryngectomy 75,
77–82
tube 72, 81
Laryngoscopy 76
Laryngo-tracheo-
bronchitis 49, 50,
65
Larynx 12, 13, 67, 76,
77, 79, 82
artificial 80
carcinoma 65
injury 65
mirror 11, 12
paralysis 65, 74
swelling 76
Leukaemia 23
Lipreading 54
Little's area 7
Lymph nodes,
cervical 44, 77
(see tonsil and
adenoid)
Lymphadenopathy 20,
29

Malaise 32
Mastoid air cells 63
Mastoidectomy 63
Mediastinitis 12, 13
Medical Social
Worker 78
Meningitis 32, 36
Metastases 75
Middle ear 18, 28, 43,
48, 62–4
Mucous
membrane 28, 32,
40, 65, 70
oedema 37, 38
Mucoperichondrial
flaps 38, 40
Muscle
crico-pharyngeus 11
respiratory 66
spasm 12, 29, 49
Myasthenia gravis 65
Myringoplasty 63
Myringotomy 48

Nasal
bleeding (see
epistaxis)

blowing 26, 35, 40,
62, 63, 81
bolster 24, 25, 35,
39, 40
cavity 9, 38
fracture 41
obstruction (see
Obstruction)
packing 2, 8, 9,
23–5, 38, 39, 40, 41
polypectomy 40
polyps 40
septal
haematoma 40
septum 9, 23, 37
sinus 23, 32, 35, 40
splint 41
submucous
resection 37
Thudicum's
speculum 9, 11
turbinate 33, 38
Nasogastric
feeding 70, 77, 79
Nasopharynx 43
Nasopharyngeal tonsil
(see Adenoid)
Nausea 46, 61
Nerve
facial 63
optic 34
Nystagmus 61

Obstruction
airway 5, 10, 41, 46,
49, 75, 76
nasal 32, 37, 38, 41
oesophageal 11, 12
upper respiratory
tract 65
Oedema 49, 65
stroma 40
Oesophageal
obstruction (see
Obstruction)
Oesophageal
speech 78, 80, 81
Oesophagoscope 13
Oesophagoscopy 13
Oesophagus 12, 77, 80
junction 80
perforation (see
Perforation)
wall 11, 14